Type 2 Diabetes - From Pathophysiology to Modern Management

Edited by Mira Siderova

Published in London, United Kingdom

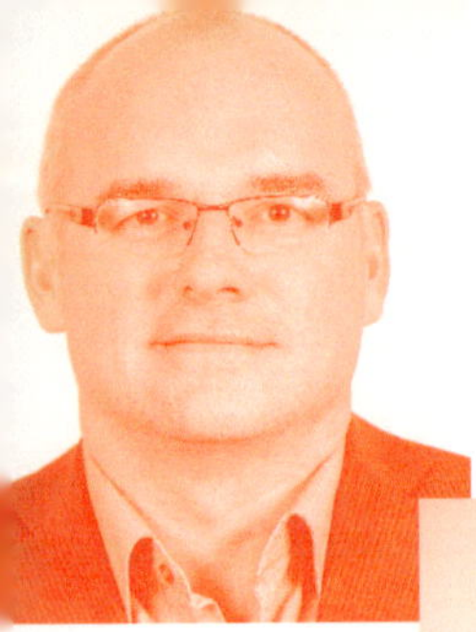
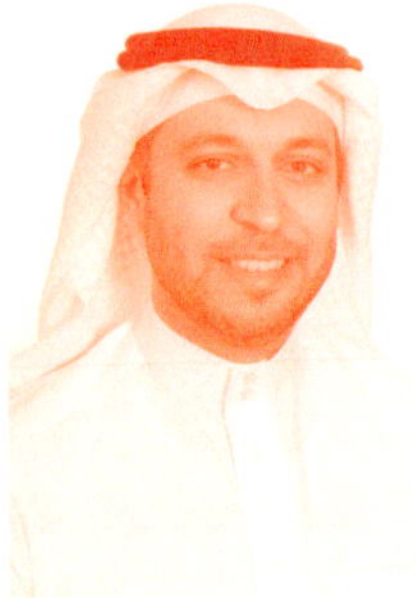
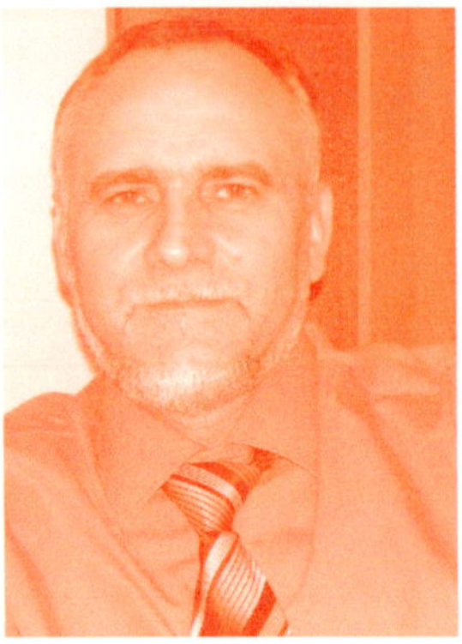
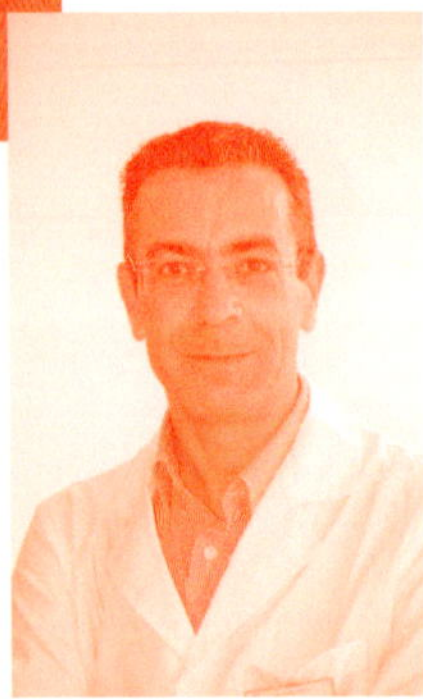
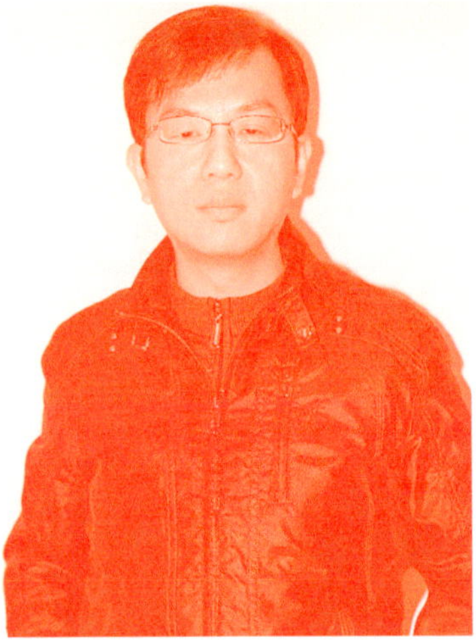
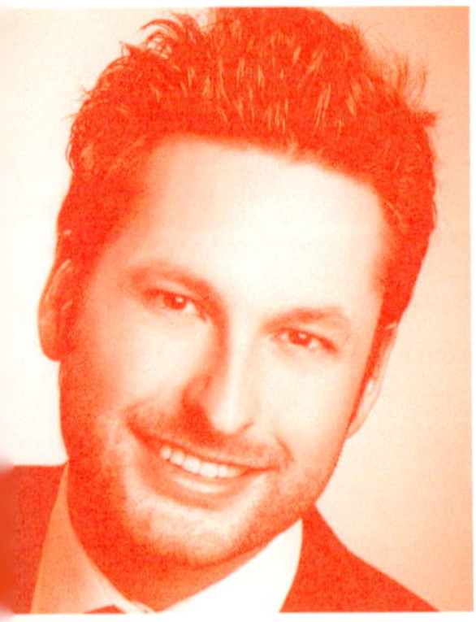
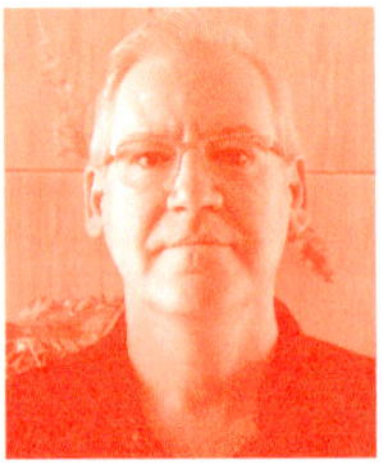

IntechOpen

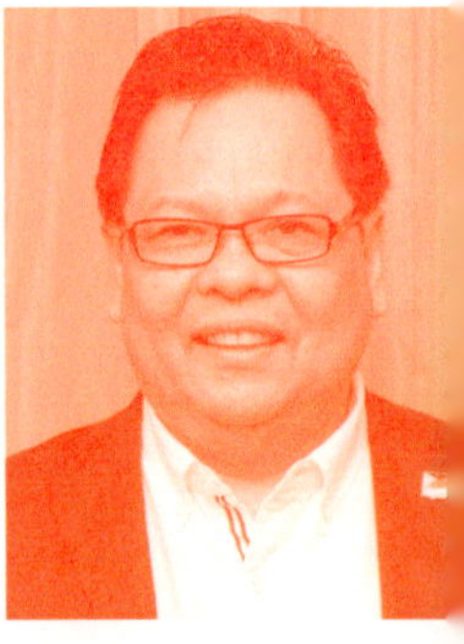
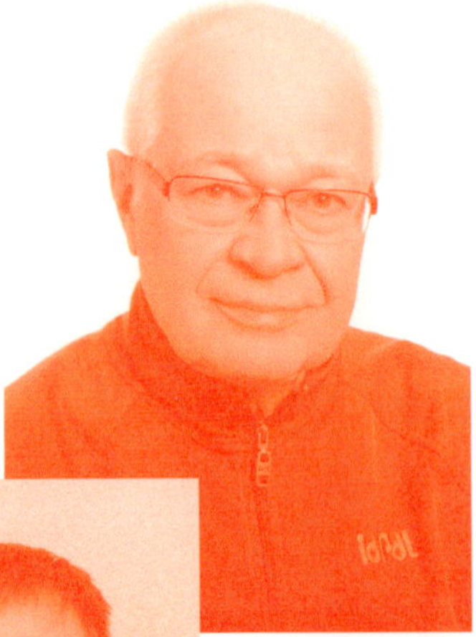
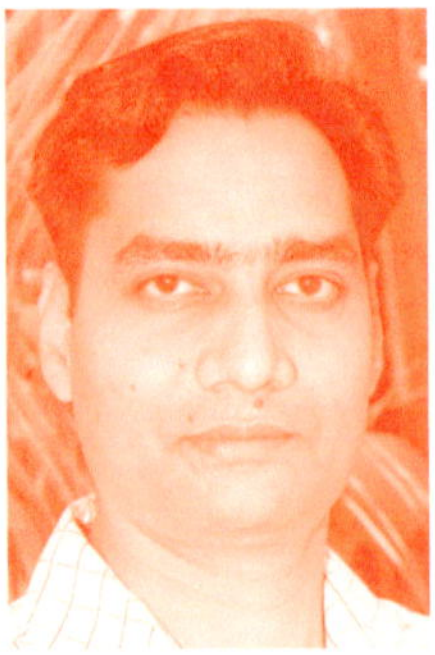
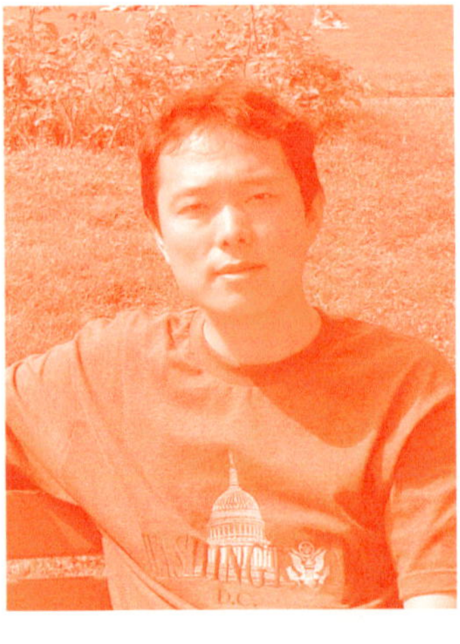
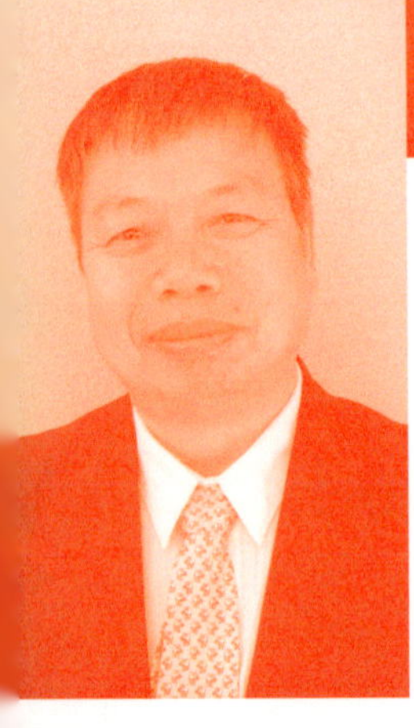
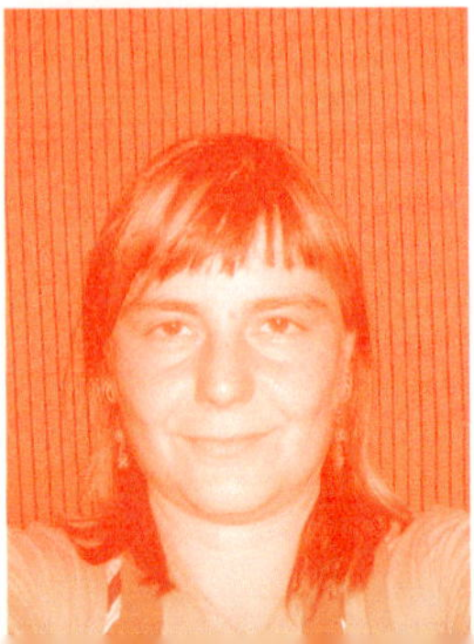

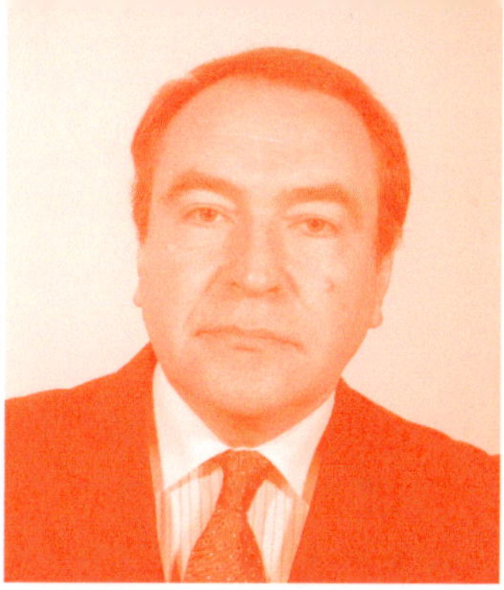

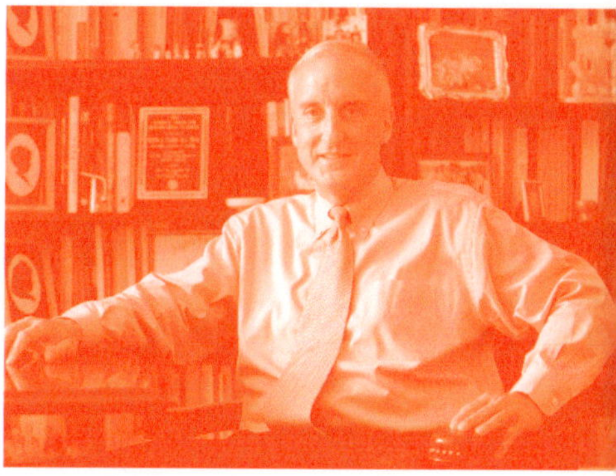

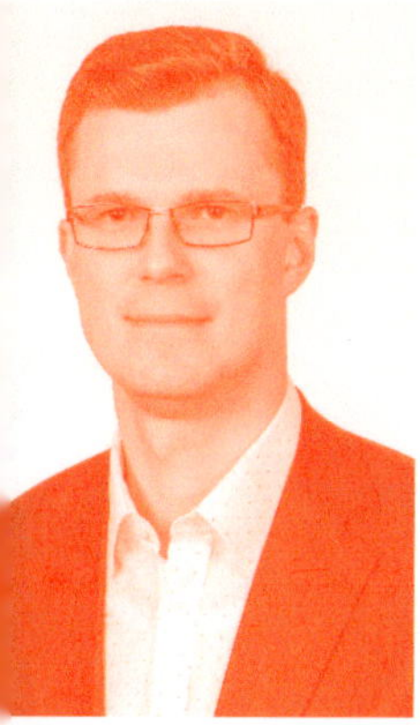

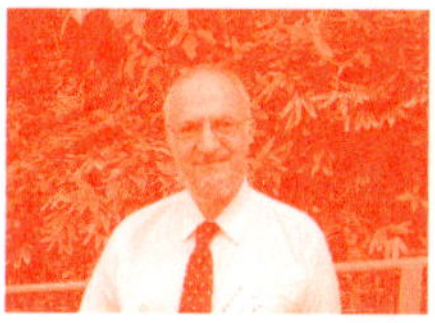

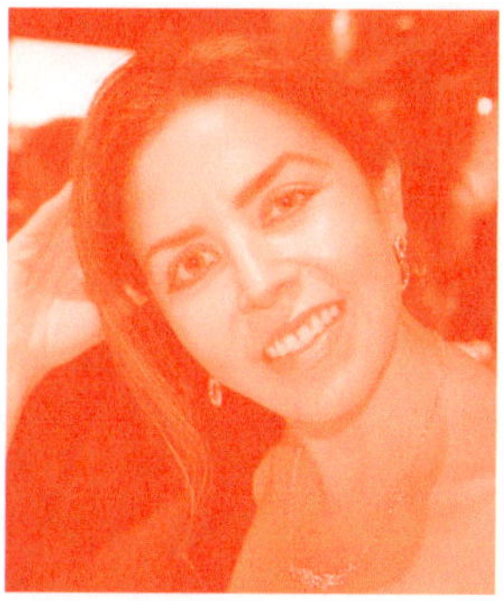

Supporting open minds since 2005

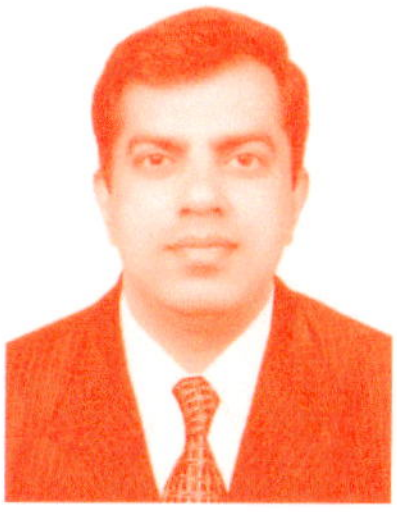

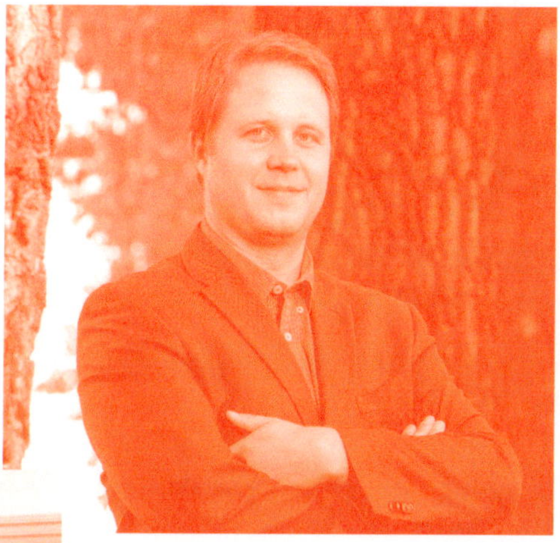

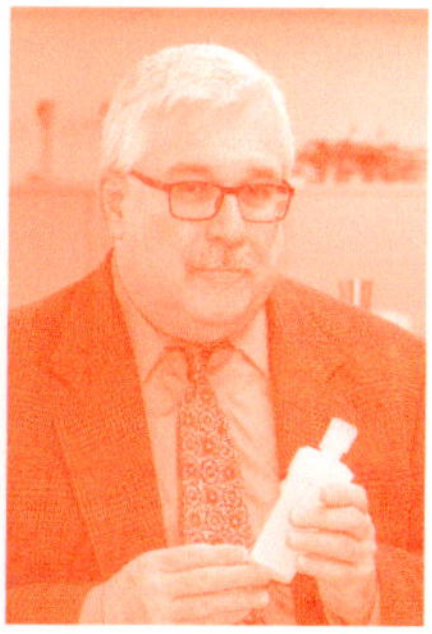

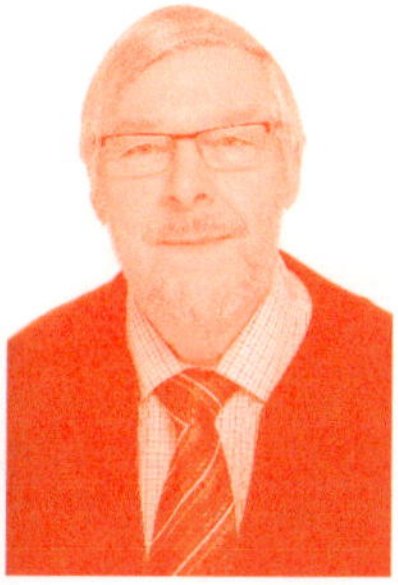

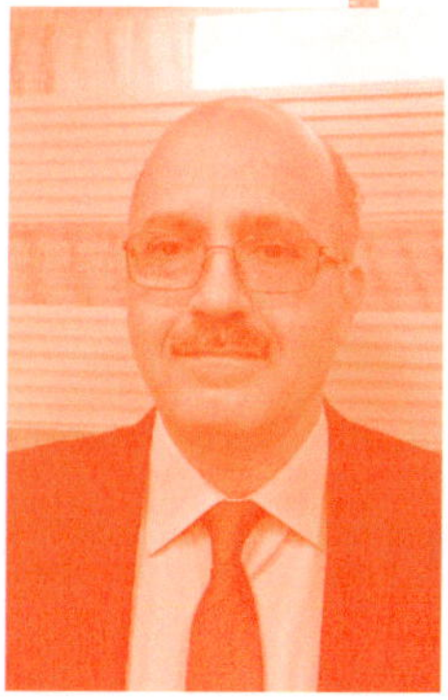

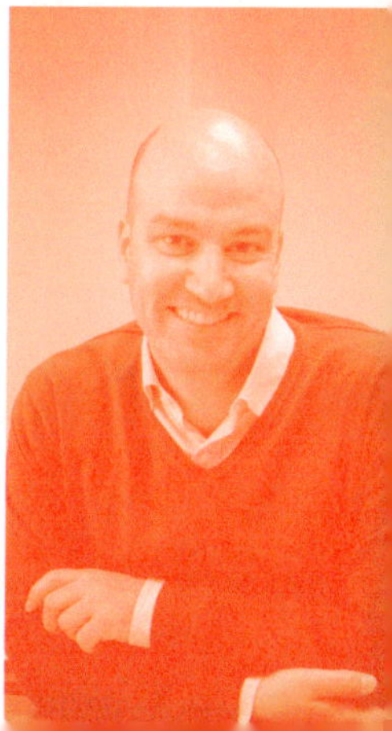

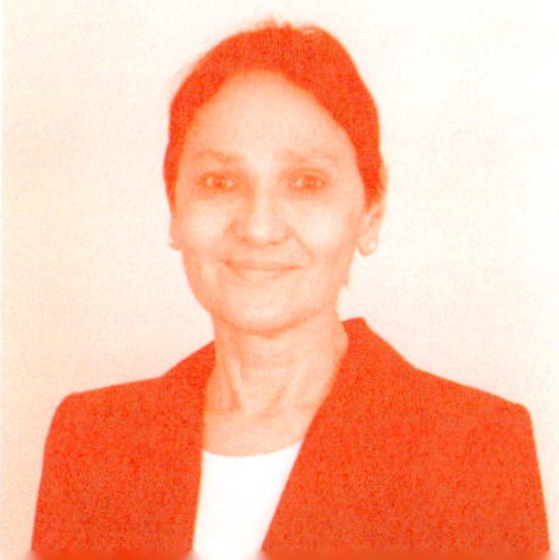

Type 2 Diabetes - From Pathophysiology to Modern Management
http://dx.doi.org/10.5772/intechopen.77683
Edited by Mira Siderova

Contributors
Alan Schorr, Pilar Durruty, Lilian Sanhueza, M.Gabriela Sanzana, Zsolt Ori, Mohammad Maswood Ahmad, Mussa Almalki, Imad Brema', Eduardo Simoes, Yilin Yoshida, Elza Tiemi Sakamoto-Hojo, Jessica Lima, Danilo Xavier, Alpana Mukhuty, Chandrani Fouzder, Snehasis Das, Dipanjan Chattopadhyay, Faiz Ahmed Shaikh, Bhuvan Kc, Thet Thet Htar, Yatinesh Kumari, Manish Gupta

First published in London, United Kingdom, 2019 by IntechOpen
IntechOpen is the global imprint of INTECHOPEN LIMITED, registered in England and Wales, registration number: 11086078, 7th floor, 10 Lower Thames Street, London, EC3R 6AF, United Kingdom
Printed in Croatia

British Library Cataloguing-in-Publication Data
A catalogue record for this book is available from the British Library

Additional hard and PDF copies can be obtained from orders@intechopen.com

Type 2 Diabetes - From Pathophysiology to Modern Management
Edited by Mira Siderova
p. cm.
Print ISBN 978-1-78923-971-3
Online ISBN 978-1-78923-972-0
eBook (PDF) ISBN 978-1-83962-914-3

For EU product safety concerns:
IN TECH d.o.o., Prolaz Marije Krucifikse Kozulić 3, 51000 Rijeka, Croatia, info@intechopen.com or visit our website at intechopen.com.

Meet the editor

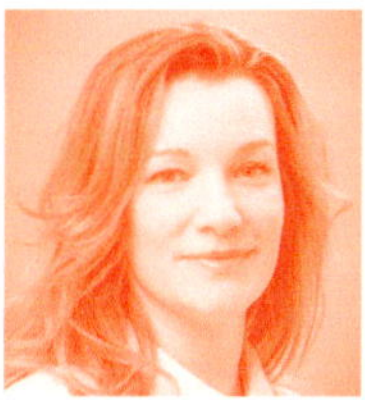

Mira Siderova, MD, PhD, is an endocrinologist at the University Hospital "St. Marina" and an Associate Professor of Endocrinology and Metabolic Diseases at the Medical University of Varna. Dr Siderova received her MD, endocrine training, and her doctorate from the Medical University of Varna and was a post-doctoral research fellow at the University of Bari, Italy. In 2015 she was awarded the prize of the Bulgarian Endocrine Society for best scientific development. She has been involved in teaching and training students, doctors, and PhD candidates in diabetes and endocrinology for the last 9 years. She has authored above 70 publications – original papers and reviews, book chapters, a monograph, and international conference reports. Her main interests are focused on diabetes, obesity, thyroid diseases, and osteoporosis. Dr Siderova is currently an independent expert at the European Commission, Research and Innovation, as well as a member of the European Thyroid Association (ETA), International Osteoporosis Federation (IOF), Bulgarian Society of Endocrinology (BDE), and Union of Scientists in Bulgaria.

Contents

Preface

The emergence of type 2 diabetes (T2D) as a global pandemic is one of the major challenges to health care in the 21st century. This book is about diabetes type 2 and it covers the newest scientific concepts in the pathogenesis of the disease as well as approaches in the diagnosis and control of diabetes and possible complications.

An important and extensively discussed topic is the progression of prediabetes to type 2 diabetes and possible lifestyle and pharmacological intervention. The role of oxidative stress, DNA damage, and DNA repair in the diabetes' progression is elucidated and the molecular impact of nutritional interventions in patients with T2D is also addressed.

The main focus of this book is glucose monitoring using cutting-edge technologies and the treatment of diabetes, especially in association with obesity. A novel cyber-physical system for management and self-management of cardiometabolic health is presented. Overall, technologies in mobile, computer, email, and internet approaches have shown evidence in enhancing chronic disease management, via supporting clinician decision-making and facilitating patient self-management among diabetic patients.

Updates on glucose lowering therapy are presented, and the new emerging class of SGLT2 inhibitors is discussed in detail. Part of the book is dedicated to the effect of diabetes on mental functions and treatment strategies to prevent cognitive decline. This book aims to contribute to the professional development of physicians, internists, endocrinologists, medical students, and research scientists in diabetes.

Mira Siderova, MD, PhD
Associate Professor,
Medical University of Varna,
University Hospital St. Marina,
Varna, Bulgaria

Section 1

Pathogenesis of Type 2 Diabetes and Its Complications

Chapter 1

Emerging Role of Pancreatic β-Cells during Insulin Resistance

Alpana Mukhuty, Chandrani Fouzder, Snehasis Das and Dipanjan Chattopadhyay

Abstract

In today's world, type 2 diabetes has become a part of every household and leads to various complications including high blood sugar level, diabetic retinopathy, diabetic foot, diabetic nephropathy and diabetic neuropathy. Yet people lack awareness about this disease and its detrimental effects. For a better understanding of this disease we must know about the causes and preventive measures since the medications used in treating type 2 diabetes have moderate to severe side effects. Type 2 diabetes is characterized by loss of insulin receptor activity in skeletal muscle and adipocytes, compensatory insulin secretion from pancreatic β-cells, β-cell dysfunction and death. The proper functioning of β-cells is a major criterion for preventing advent of type 2 diabetes. The different natural or physiological insulin secretagogues include glucose, amino acids and fatty acids, which stimulate insulin secretion under the influence of various hormones like incretins, leptin, growth hormone, melatonin and estrogen. However, excess of nutrients lead to β-cell dysfunction and dearth of insulin involving various signal molecules like SIRT1, PPARγ, TLR4, NF-KB, Wnt, mTOR, inflammasomes, MCP1, EGFR, and Nrf2. A deeper insight into the functioning of these signaling molecules will also create new avenues for therapeutic interventions of curing β-cell dysfunction and death.

Keywords: insulin resistance, pancreatic β-cell dysfunction, lipotoxicity, glucotoxicity, type 2 diabetes

1. Introduction

Changing food habits, sedentary lifestyle and obesity has made type 2 diabetes (T2D) a global epidemic. T2D has various characteristic features such as insulin resistance caused when peripheral tissues such as liver, muscle and adipocytes have a decreased response to insulin. The progression from normal glucose tolerance to type 2 diabetes involves several transitional stages of impaired fasting glucose and impaired glucose tolerance which is known as prediabetes. The mechanism leading to the development of these glucose metabolic alterations is multifactorial. The most prevalent factor of T2D is insulin resistance that occurs when peripheral tissues such as liver, muscle and adipocytes, the main target organs of Insulin hormone, loses the ability to respond to insulin [1]. Generally in the obese patients without T2D and initially in people who develop insulin resistance, pancreatic β-cells are able to compensate for insulin resistance by increasing insulin secretion by increasing β-cell mass via increased proliferation and hypertrophy [2, 3].

Increasing of β-cells in a compensatory mechanism to avoid the complications caused due to insulin resistance and henceforth prevents diabetes [4]. This unique mechanism of β-cell mass expansion has been observed in normal individuals during physiological growth [5] as well as in insulin resistant patients, especially pregnant women [6] and obese people [7]. In patients having T2D the initial stage of β-cell compensation is followed by dysfunction or failure of β-cells due to less proliferation and increased apoptosis [1, 8].

Pancreatic β-cell dysfunction plays a critical role in progression of T2D. Insulin is produced as preproinsulin and then processed to proinsulin. Proinsulin is then converted to insulin and C-peptide and stored in secretory granules. Synthesis of insulin is regulated at both transcription and translational level. Several transcription factors in the cis-acting sequences within the 5′ region and trans-activators regulate insulin gene transcription. These transcription factors are paired homeobox gene 6 (PAX6), pancreatic and duodenal homeobox-1 (Pdx-1), MafA and B-2/Neurogenic differentiation 1 (NeuroD1). Insulin secretion from β-cells contains a series of events and is controlled by variety of factors and signaling pathways that ultimately leads to the fusion of secretory granules with the plasma membrane. The various stimulants that regulate insulin secretion are glucose, free fatty acids, amino acids, also various hormones like melatonin, estrogen, leptin, growth hormone and glucagon like peptide-1 [9].

2. Structure of insulin

The monomeric structure of insulin is made up of "A" chain with 21 amino acids and "B" chain with 30 amino acids, which are bound by disulfide bonds. Actually three disulfide bonds are present in the structure of insulin monomer, two in between the A and B chains (A7–B7, A20–B19) and one within the A chain (A7–A11) [10]. The secondary structure of the A chain is made up of two anti-parallel α-helices in between A2–A8 and A13–A19 residues. Also the helices are connected by residues at A9–A12. As a result of this particular arrangement the two ends remains in close proximity to each other and side by side [11].

The B chain is made up of α-helices and β-pleated sheets [11] and in the T state it exists in two different conformations in crystallized form [12]. The α-helix exists between B9 and B19, a β-turn between B20 and B23 and the chain folds in a "V" due to Gly20 and Gly23. An extended β-strand structure in between residues B24 and B30 which allows the chain to be in close proximity to form a β-sheet with PheB24 and TyrB26 which are in close contact with B11 and B15 leucine residues of α-helix. There is a continuous α-helix from B1 to B19 in the R state. The stability of the native insulin structure is due to the disulfide bonds in between Cys residues A7–B7 and A20–B19. The affinity of insulin towards the insulin receptor is determined by the side chain interactions in between A chain and B chain. These disulfide bonds between the A and B chain provide the tertiary structure of insulin monomer which is very highly organized. The various amino acid interactions in the side chain also contribute to the stable tertiary structure of the insulin monomer molecule. These interactions are also responsible for the interaction or affinity of insulin towards its receptor [11].

The hydrophobic inner core of the insulin monomer is composed of the following amino acids residues: A6–A11 and Leu A11, B1 and B15, Ile A2, Phe B24, Val A3, Ile A13, Val B18 and Val B12. The amino acid residues from B20 to B23 are necessary for stabilizing the β-turn thereby leading to the folding of the β-sheet in between B23 and B30 towards the α-helix and hydrophobic inner core. In the dimeric form of insulin these non-polar amino acids remain in the inner side. The insulin subunits

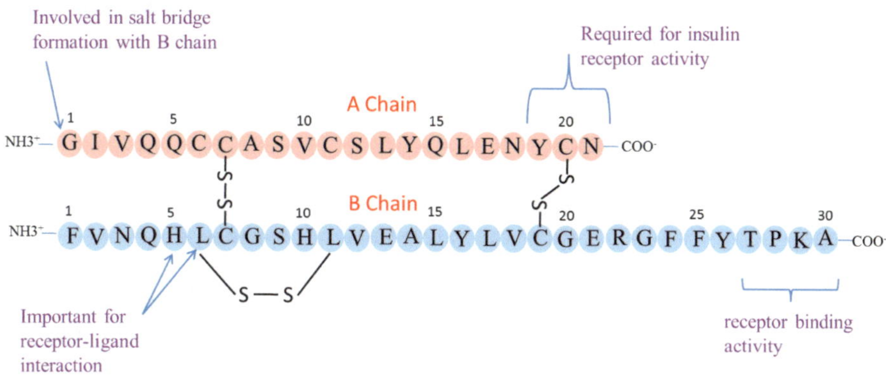

Figure 1.
Structure of insulin [10, 11, 12, 20].

generally remain as dimers [12]. The dimeric form of insulin is stabilized by the antiparallel β-sheets at the carboxy terminals of the B chains which remain expose on the surface of the dimeric structure. The hydrophobic core of the insulin dimer is composed of non-polar residues [11].

There are three dimers made up of six molecules of insulin peptide to make a hexamer. Some differences in the side chain like in the 25th residue (Phe) in the B chain, which is arranged to be inside the hydrophobic core of the peptide chain on one side of the dimer, deforms the perfect two-fold symmetry [11]. Also there are two zinc atoms with the imidazole groups in three histidine residues in the B chain along with two water molecules in the insulin hexamer [12].

The knowledge about the structure of insulin is necessary to understand its interaction with insulin receptor. The amino acids in the specific regions of the insulin molecule that facilitate its binding with the receptor are located at the amino terminal of the A chain: GlyA1, IleA2, ValA3, GluA4: carboxy terminal of the A chain: TyrA19, CysA20, AsnA21; and carboxy terminal of the B chain: GlyB23, PheB24, PheB25, TyrB26. These residues have are denoted as the "cooperative site" of the insulin due to their negative cooperativity [13, 14].

- Out of the two chains in the structure of insulin, the A chain has more significant role for binding to the receptor. Acetylation of the amino terminal reduces binding to receptor by 30% which makes a free amino terminus necessary for binding to receptor [15].

- Gly1 deletion reduces binding to receptor by 15% which may be due to some salt bridge formation between Gly1 and B chain carboxy terminus [16].

- Also TyrA19, CysA20 and AsnA21 in the carboxy terminus of the A chain are also necessary for insulin receptor activity [16].

- The carboxy terminal of the B chain has also a significant role in the receptor binding activity, specially the first four residues, whose deletion reduces receptor binding activity by 30% [17, 18].

- Fifteen percent of the receptor binding activity is detained when HisB5 is deleted and 1% of binding activity is reduced when LeuB6 is deleted [19].

- For the maintenance of disulfide bonds between A and B chain, CysB7 is critical [20].

- HisB10 is necessary for activity because when substituted with AspB10, proinsulin is not converted to insulin [21].
- However, synthetic insulin containing AspB10 has 500% greater binding affinity than normal insulin [22].
- PheB24 forms hydrogen bonds important for dimer formation and PheB25 is important for conformation of the native insulin structure [16].
- GlyB23, PheB24, PheB25 and TyrB26 in the B chain carboxy terminus are evolutionarily conserved residues needed for receptor binding [16] (**Figure 1**).

3. Insulin synthesis

The various stimulants in blood that lead to insulin secretion are glucose, monosaccharide, amino acid and fatty acid.

3.1 Glucose stimulated insulin secretion

Glucose acts as the main stimulus for insulin secretion in rodents as well as human beings because it is one of the major constituents of their diet and enters the circulation immediately after digestion of food. Glucose transporter 2, i.e., GLUT2 is the main glucose sensor found in the plasma membrane of β-cells. Translocation of GLUT2 to plasma membrane is dependent on insulin and it bears low substrate affinity, hence leading to high uptake of glucose. Upon entry into β-cell glucose is phosphorylated to glucose-6-phosphate by glucokinase, a type of hexokinase. Glucokinase is the rate-limiting step in the glucose metabolism in β-cells [23]. Since pyruvate dehydrogenase is not found in β-cells, pyruvate is metabolized to produce metabolic coupling factors via two pathways: (a) pyruvate is metabolized to acetyl-coA and thereby it enters glucose oxidation: the main signaling pathway couple to pyruvate oxidation through the tricarboxylic acid cycle (TCA) by mitochondria "ATP-sensitive potassium (K_{ATP}) channel-dependent insulin release." The other pathway is anaplerosis where pyruvate, like other TCA cycle intermediates is replenished. However, some of the products of these processes can act as signals stimulating release of insulin, like malonyl-CoA, NADPH, and glutamate. These products are known to amplify K_{ATP} channel-dependent insulin secretion [24, 25].

Formation of glycerol-3-phosphate (Gly3P) is the third glucose signal. Glucokinase phosphorylates glucose into glucose-6-phosphate (G6P), G6P then enters glycolysis to produce pyruvate. Gly3P can also be produced by G6P via dihydroxyacetone phosphate (DHAP) pathway. These compounds stimulate insulin secretion. Gly3P also promotes β-cell glycolysis via the mitochondrial Gly3P NADH shuttle process, which activates mitochondrial energy metabolism and augments insulin secretion [26, 27]. Dysfunction of β-cells after prolonged exposure to elevated levels of glucose has been linked to changes in glucose detection and metabolism, apoptosis, and calcium handling. Now it has already been reported that glucotoxicity impedes final steps in insulin secretion, i.e., exocytosis [28].

3.2 Fatty acids and insulin secretion

Free fatty acids (FFAs) exert both positive and negative effects on β-cell survival and insulin secretory function, depending on concentration, duration, and glucose abundance. Insulin secretion from β-cell is also stimulated by free fatty acids (FFAs).

The FFAs can also upregulate glucose stimulated insulin secretion (GSIS) from β-cells. In total absence of FFAs the β-cells lose their insulin secreting capability which can again be restored when exogenous fatty acids are added [29–31]. The FFAs act upon β-cells through free fatty acid receptor (FFAR)-1, hence controlling β-cell function [32, 33]. The intracellular metabolism of FFA leads to the production of lipid signal molecules like long-chain acyl-CoA and DAG [34]. DAG in turn activates protein kinase C (PKC), which in turn tales part in insulin secretion [35]. The effect of fatty acids on pancreatic islet insulin release depends mainly on degree and time of exposure. Circulating low levels of free fatty acids in the range of physiologic postprandial values actually aids in enhancing glucose-induced insulin secretion. However, excessive accumulation of lipids within islets impairs insulin secretion [36].

3.3 Amino acid stimulated insulin secretion

At individual concentrations amino acids found in physiological concentrations are poor insulin secretagogues. Some combinations of amino acids at physiological concentrations are capable of enhancing GSIS [37], like that of, glutamine cannot stimulate insulin secretion or enhance GSIS alone, but in combination with leucine, glutamine is capable of stimulating insulin secretion from β-cells and enhancing GSIS [38]. Leucine activates glutamate dehydrogenase, and glutamate dehydrogenase can convert glutamate to α-ketoglutarate, leading to production of ATP and stimulating insulin secretion [37]. Two important incretin hormones secreted from K-cells and L-cells in the gastrointestinal tract, Glucose dependent insulinotropic peptide (GIP) and glucagon-like peptide-1 (GLP-1), are stimulated to be secreted after ingestion of nutrients like glucose and amino acids. These hormone levels rise in the circulation after feeding food rich in protein and carbohydrates. Then they directly trigger insulin secretion from β-cells by binding to their specific cell-surface receptors, hence enhancing GSIS [39–41].

4. Regulation of insulin secretion

4.1 Neural and hormone regulation

4.1.1 GLP-1

GLP-1 is an incretin hormone secreted from small intestinal L-cells along with GIP when the nutrient content in blood is high generally after ingestion [42, 43]. Nutrient load from oral route triggers more insulin secretion than intravenous nutrient load [44]. GLP1-agonists and analogues are already used as an effective therapy for type 2 diabetes that are safe due to the glucose dependent effect on the insulin secretion and large randomized clinical trials proved their additional cardiovascular benefits [45]. GLP-1 acts upon β-cells due to the presence of GLP-1 receptor (GLP-1R). Activation of GLP-1R leads to activation of adenylyl cyclase, which in turn generates cAMP. Elevated level of cAMP in the cytosol enhances GSIS. Hence GLP-1 secretion is dependent on high blood glucose levels [45, 46].

4.1.2 Leptin

Leptin, secreted from adipocytes, regulates function of insulin upon the glucose storing fat and liver cells [47, 48]. However, in absence of leptin, hyperinsulinemia leads to drop in blood glucose levels [47, 49]. The inhibitory action of leptin has been well known in clonal β-cells [50], cultured rodent islets [51], perfused rodent pancreas [50, 52], human islets [51, 53, 54] and mice islets [51]. Leptin inhibits insulin secretion by antagonizing the action of elevated intracellular cAMP [55]. 3-isobutyl-1-methylxanthine (IBMX) induces leptin, elevating cAMP content by inhibiting phosphodiesterases (PDEs) [56], the enzymes which catalyze hydrolysis of cAMP. GLP-1-induced insulin secretion is also inhibited by leptin, and GLP-1 which augments insulin secretion by activation of the cAMP signaling pathways [52].

4.1.3 Estrogen

In the "classical" mechanism of action of estrogen, the estrogen molecules diffuse into cell and bind to the estrogen receptor ER located in the nucleus. Rapid or "nongenomic" effects of estrogen are thought to occur through the ER located in or adjacent to the plasma membrane and may require presence of "adaptor" proteins, which target the ER to the membrane. Activation of the membrane ER leads to a rapid change in cellular signaling molecules and stimulation of kinase activity, which in turn may affect transcription [57].

β-cells are not general estrogen targets but the presence of estrogen receptor in islets makes the effect of 17β-estradiol on β-cells noteworthy [58, 59]. 17β-estradiol enhances insulin secretion from β-cells [60] and in humans, it is known to increase insulin secretion in postmenopausal women [61, 62], thus it augments glucose-stimulated insulin secretion (GSIS) [63]. Two types of are present in β-cells: (1) the estrogen receptors in the nucleus, i.e., nuclear ERs (ERα and ERβ) and (2) the estrogen receptors in the membrane, i.e., the membrane ER (ERγ) [64]. 17β-estradiol significantly decreases activity of K_{ATP} channel [60], causing membrane depolarization and opening of voltage-gated Ca^{2+} channels, thereby potentiating glucose-induced intracellular [Ca^{2+}] oscillations, in a reversible manner.

4.1.4 Melatonin

Melatonin, a hormone secreted by pineal gland, helps in maintaining circadian rhythm and biological clock [65]. However, melatonin receptors are found on clonal β-cells [66, 67] and human islets [68]. Melatonin shows both stimulatory [69] and inhibitory effects [70, 71], as well as neutral effects [72] on insulin section. However a decent number of reports have been found in literature about the inhibitory effect of melatonin in clonal β-cells [66, 68, 69, 73]. Melatonin inhibits glucose- and KCl-stimulated insulin secretion in rat islets [74]. Long term melatonin administration enhances hyperinsulinemia in vivo [75]. The signaling pathway of melatonin shows that melatonin receptor is coupled to Gi, which inhibits G protein [76]. Melatonin mediates stimulatory effect on insulin secretion through its receptor MTNR1A, by activation of Gq/11 which provokes release of IP3 by activating PLC-ε to augment insulin secretion [69, 77, 78].

4.1.5 Growth hormone

Growth hormone (GH) stimulates production of insulin-like growth factor-I (IGF-I) and its binding proteins [79]. Human IGF1 and IGF2 show high sequence similarity with insulin. Insulin receptor (IR) has two isoforms, IRA and IRB. IRB only binds insulin with high affinity while IRA binds both insulin and IGF2 with equal affinity. The IGF1 receptor (IGF1R) has high affinity towards both IGF1 and IGF2 but it binds insulin with very low affinity. According to the conventional view regarding the actions of insulin and IGF-1 in mammals, insulin mediates mainly a metabolic response, and IGF-1 mediates growth promoting effects in vivo [80]. Recombinant human IGF-I decreases serum levels of insulin and C-peptide in human [81]. IGF-1 also suppresses insulin secretion in isolated rat islets [82]. This inhibitory activity of growth hormone is mediated through PDE3B activation [83], which is responsible for breaking down cAMP in β-cells.

4.1.6 Adrenergic and cholinergic agents

Adrenergic drugs (epinephrine, norepinephrine and isoproterenol) are known to inhibit insulin secretion by binding to alpha receptors present in rat pancreas. On the other hand cholinergic drugs (acetylcholine and carbamylcholine) stimulate insulin secretion but this effect is suppressed by simultaneous addition of atropine. Thus the autonomic nervous system regulates insulin secretion under physiological conditions [84] (**Figure 2**).

4.2 Regulation by signaling pathways

4.2.1 SIRT1

SIRT1, mammalian sirtuin homolog, plays a key role in energy homeostasis and extends a cell lifespan by calorie restriction [85]. Glucose metabolism is tightly coupled to the regulation of insulin secretion and β-cell function [86]. Till now there are two reports showing SIRT1 positively regulates glucose-stimulated insulin secretion in pancreatic β-cells [87, 88]. In β-cells, FoxO1 is constitutively phosphorylated in cytoplasm, and activates insulin receptor signaling [89]. Accumulation of FoxO1 in the nucleus of insulin-secreting cells is triggered by palmitate during induction of lipotoxicity and impairs insulin secretion [90, 91]. Increased expression of SIRT1 in pancreatic β cells in mice improves glucose tolerance by enhancing insulin secretion [87]; deletion of SIRT1 can impair glucose-stimulated insulin secretion [88]. In both these reports, SIRT1 enhances insulin secretion by transcriptional repression of uncoupling protein 2 (UCP2) [92]. Activation of SIRT1 gives

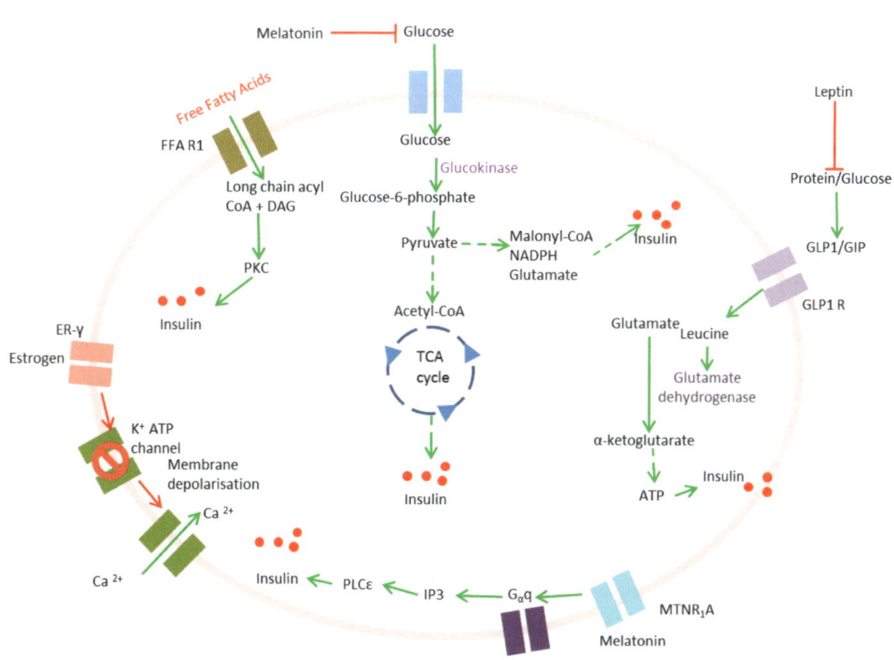

Figure 2.
Hormonal and nutrient regulation of insulin secretion [23, 26, 27, 32–35, 45, 46, 55, 57, 60, 64, 72].

protection from high-fat-induced obesity and insulin resistance [92–94], and slight overexpression of SIRT1 has a protective role from high-fat induced glucose intolerance [95–97]. If SIRT1 is inhibited then insulin promoter activity is suppressed, insulin regulatory genes such as v-maf musculoaponeurotic fibrosarcoma oncogene homolog A (MafA) and NK6 homeodomain 1 (NKX6.1) mRNA expressions are down regulated leading to decreased insulin secretion. On the contrary, activation or overexpression of SIRT1 antagonizes reduced insulin transcriptional activity by exerting negative effect on pancreatic and duodenal homeobox 1 (PDX1)-stimulated insulin promoter activity and also abolishes forkhead box O1 protein (FOXO1)-insulin transcriptional activity [98].

4.2.2 PPARγ

PPAR-γ regulates the major β cell genes involved in glucose sensing, insulin secretion and insulin gene transcription and protects from glucose, lipid, cytokine and islet amyloid polypeptide (IAPP)-induced stress pathways [99]. PPAR-γ is a member of nuclear hormone receptor superfamily of ligand-activated transcription factors and TZDs are oral agents that are high-affinity activators of PPAR-γ [100]. PPARγ ablation protects mice from high fat diet induced insulin resistance [101] and isolated islets from these mice show blunted TZD response towards GSIS [102]. Mice with PPAR-γ ablated pancreas show glucose intolerance at baseline with downregulated Pdx-1 and GLUT2 expression in their isolated islets [103]. Chronic high glucose can decrease PPAR-γ mRNA levels in mouse islets [104]. PPAR-γ is upregulated after 60% pancreatectomy procedure in rats changing to pro differentiation state from proliferative state [105]. Promoters of GLUT2 and glucokinase have functional PPREs that bind PPAR-γ/RXRα heterodimer, and lead to transcriptional upregulation of these genes in β cell [106, 107]. The expression of these genes is impaired in diabetic rodent models [108, 109].

PPARγ agonists modulate IAPP-induced ER stress [110]. The islet-specific KO of the ATP-binding membrane cassette transporter protein A1 (ABCA1) and PPAR-γ KO model both show increased intra-islet triglyceride accumulation and lowered GSIS [101, 111]. Rosiglitazone restores GSIS and decreases apoptosis in isolated human lipotoxic islets with a reduction in intra-islet triglyceride accumulation and reduced inducible nitric oxide synthase (iNOS) expression [112, 113]. PPAR-γ agonists also inhibit cytokine-induced activation of JNK in insulinoma cell lines [114]. PPAR-γ agonists have been shown to increase AKT phosphorylation in the setting of both IAPP-and lipid-inducted toxicity. These effects were blocked by PI3 kinase inhibitors and associated with increased levels of insulin receptor substrate 2 (IRS2) proteins [115].

Activation of PPAR-γ inhibits IL-1β and IFN-γ stimulated nuclear translocation of p65 subunit of NF-KB and DNA binding activity leading to reduced inducible nitric oxide synthase and cyclooxygenase-2 expression [116].

PPAR-γ activation also increases intracellular calcium mobilization, insulin secretion, and β-cell gene expression through GPR40 and GLUT2 gene upregulation [117]. Thus PPAR-γ agonists not only improve insulin sensitivity in the target tissues, but also act within the β-cells.

4.2.3 Wnt

Wnt signaling stimulates β-cell proliferation, specifically Wnt3a promotes expression of Pitx2, a direct target of Wnt signaling, and Cyclin D2, an essential regulator of cell cycle progression [118]. Single nucleotide polymorphisms (SNPs) in TCF7L2 are linked to etiology of T2D [119]. Expression of three Tcf genes

(Tcf7, Tcf7l1, Tcf7l2) in pancreas is reduced by treatment with insulin or high fat diet feeding [120]. A significant elevation of TCF7L2 mRNA expression occurs in pancreatic islets along with impaired insulin secretion [121]. TCF7L2 depletion in isolated human or mouse pancreatic islets results in significant increased β-cell apoptosis and decreased proliferation with attenuated GSIS. Over-expression of TCF7L2 protects islets from glucose- and cytokine-mediated apoptosis [122]. These findings suggest that β-cell function and survival are positively regulated by the expression of Tcf7l2 in type 2 diabetes.

4.2.4 mTOR

Rapamycin, an mTORC1 complex inhibitor, reduces the number and proliferation of pancreatic and endocrine progenitors. Mice lacking mTOR in pancreatic progenitors suffer from hyperglycemia in neonates, hypoinsulinemia and pancreatic agenesis/hypoplasia with pancreas rudiments containing ductal structures lacking differentiated acinar and endocrine cells [123].

AMP-activated protein kinase (AMPK) is a controller of β-cell function. Inhibition of AMPK in β-cells by high glucose inversely correlates with activation of the mammalian Target of Rapamycin (mTOR) pathway. Glucose and amino acid sensing ability of AMPK is important in regulation of insulin secretion [124]. Rapamycin also induces fulminant diabetes by increasing insulin resistance and reducing-cell function and mass [125].

Obesity induced by excess nutrient intake leads to the upregulation of mTORC1/S6K1 signaling in insulin-sensitive tissues, including β-cells [126–128]. mTORC1 activation play an initial role in adaptation to nutrient excess and obesity, but chronic and persistent hyperactivation could lead to development of insulin resistance by a negative feedback loop on IRS signaling [129].

4.2.5 MCP1

Monocyte chemoattractant protein-1 (MCP-1) a chemokine that regulates migration and infiltration of monocytes/macrophages, is constitutively present in normal human islet β-cells in the absence of an inflammatory infiltrate and plays a key role in monocyte recruitment [130]. NF-kappaB plays an important role for MCP-1 expression in β-cells [131]. MCP-1 also induces amylin expression through ERK1/2/JNK-AP1 and NF-κB related signaling pathways independent of CCR2. Amylin upregulation by MCP-1 may contribute to elevation of plasma amylin in obesity and insulin resistance [132].

4.2.6 Nrf2

The Keap1-Nrf2 signaling plays an important role in oxidative stress response and metabolism. Nrf2 prevents reactive oxygen species ROS mediated damage in pancreatic β-cells [133]. β-cells have low expression levels of antioxidant enzymes, making them susceptible to damage caused by ROS. GLP-1 effectively inhibits oxidative stress and cell death of β-cells induced by the pro-oxidant tert-butyl hydroperoxide (tert-BOOH) [134]. NOX activation through Src signaling plays an important role in ROS overproduction and impaired GSIS caused by lipotoxicity [135].

4.2.7 EGFR

Epidermal growth factor receptors are crucial regulators of β-cell proliferation and β-cell mass regulation. Partial tissue-specific attenuation of EGFR signaling in islets leads to significantly reduced beta-cell proliferation [136]. Phosphorylation of ribosomal S6 kinase, a mammalian target of rapamycin (mTOR) target, is upregulated in islets from glucose and interleukin injected 6-month-old rats. β-cell mass expansion occurs in presence of chronic nutrient excess EGFR signaling, mTOR activation, and FOXM1-mediated cell proliferation [137].

4.2.8 ER stress

In pancreatic β-cells, the endoplasmic reticulum (ER) is an important cellular compartment involved in insulin biosynthesis. ER stress elicits a signaling cascade known as the unfolded protein response (UPR) which regulates both function and survivability of β-cells [138]. Chronic high glucose leads to insulin mRNA degradation by IRE1α activation, profuse XBP-1 splicing, and induction of pro-apoptotic effectors, such as Jun N-terminal kinase (JNK) and C/EBP homologous protein (CHOP), causing β-cell dysfunction and death [139–142]. Free fatty acids (FFAs) and inflammatory cytokines also induce ER stress in β-cells through upregulation of the proapoptotic effector CHOP, and JNK and caspase-12 activation by UPR [143–146].

4.2.9 Inflammasome

ER stress, oxidative stress and high glucose concentrations activates NLRP3 inflammasome leading to interleukin (IL)-1β production and caspase-1 dependent pyroptosis. Whether IL-1β or intrinsic NLRP3 inflammasome activation contributes to β-cell death is disputed [147].

The Nlrp3 inflammasome plays important role in obesity-induced insulin resistance and β-cell failure. Endocannabinoids contribute to insulin resistance through activation of peripheral CB_1 receptors (CB_1Rs) promoting β-cell failure [148]. *NLRP3*-knockout mice showed improved glucose profiles after a high-fat diet, due to attenuated IL-1β release from islet cells. Hyperglycemia-induced IL-1β release leads to increased ROS, dissociation of TXNIP from thioredoxin and its binding to NLRP3 and activation of NLRP3 [149].

4.2.10 TLR4

Toll-like receptor 4 (TLR4), a pattern recognition receptor, is a crucial element in the triggering of innate immunity, which binds to pathogen-associated molecules such as Lipopolysaccharide (LPS), and initiates a cascade of pro-inflammatory events [150]. TLR4 is also known to occur in pancreatic β-cells but its function is yet to be clearly established. β-cells respond to palmitate via TLR4/MyD88 pathway and produce chemokines that recruit M1-type proinflammatory monocytes/macrophages to the islets [151]. High fat diet-induced obesity stimulates TLR4 up-regulation in pancreatic β-cells, and lead to the recruitment of macrophage into pancreatic islet, which finally results in pancreatic β-cell dysfunction [152].

Fetuin-A, a secreted glycoprotein, can promote lipotoxicity in β-cells through the TLR4-JNK-NF-κB signaling pathway [153]. Later it was also discovered that pancreatic β-cells are capable of secreting fetuin-A under free fatty acid stimulation which ultimately leads to inflammation [154].

4.2.11 G-proteins

Medium- to long-chain fatty acids activate FFAR1/GPR40 and it is predominantly coupled to $G\alpha_q$ which signals through PLC-mediated hydrolysis of

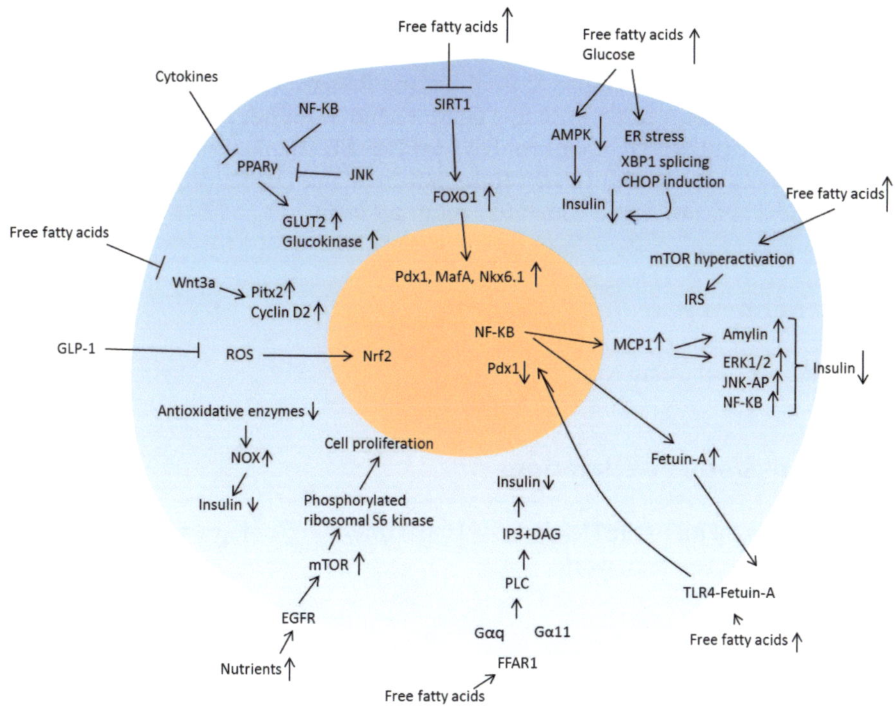

Figure 3.
Various signaling pathways regulating insulin secretion signaling [90, 91, 98, 99, 106, 107, 120, 129, 132, 134, 135, 137, 139–142, 153–157].

membrane phospholipids leading to the formation of IP_3 and DAG [155, 156]. Glucose tolerance and insulin secretion is impaired in mice due to β-cell-specific inactivation of the genes encoding the G protein α-subunits $G\alpha_q$ and $G\alpha_{11}$. Thus, G_q/G_{11}-mediated signaling pathway mediates insulin secretion by glucose stimulation [157] (**Figure 3**).

5. Conclusion

In conclusion, insulin secretion is stimulated by glucose, free fatty acids and amino acids after their breakdown in gut following ingestion. Glucose potentiates K_{ATP} channel-dependent insulin secretion. Free fatty acids result in insulin secretion from β-cells through free fatty acid receptor (FFAR)-1. Under incretin stimulation the amino acids trigger insulin secretion by binding to their cell surface receptors. Hormones like GLP-1 and estrogen stimulate insulin secretion, melatonin has both stimulatory and inhibitory effect and leptin and growth hormone have only inhibitory effects upon insulin secretion. Discussing about the various signaling pathways, mainly Wnt, G-proteins, EGFR, mTOR, SIRT1, PPARγ mediate increased insulin secretion, β-cell proliferation and improved GSIS in presence of nutrients, while in case of excessive nutrient load TLR4, MCP1, inflammasomes and Nrf2 impairs insulin secretion and conduces β-cell death. These excess of nutrients are the key players behind glucotoxicity and lipotoxicity, which ultimately lead to compensatory insulin secretion, β-cell mass expansion initially and β-cell death under chronic nutrients overload. Our major concern should be leading a healthy lifestyle, active routine, regular exercise, balanced diet and constant awareness about the incidence of type 2 diabetes, for eradication and curing of the disease to some extent.

Acknowledgements

AM is thankful to the Science & Engineering Research Board (SERB), Department of Science & Technology, Govt. of India, for her JRF fellowship (Grant No. ECR/2017/001028). DC thankful DBT for JRF. SD thanks UGC, New Delhi for SRF. The authors are thankful to Dr. Rakesh Kundu and Dr. Sandip Mukherjee for their technical assistance and constant encouragement.

Conflict of interest

The authors declare no conflict of interest.

Notes/thanks/other declarations

The authors thank to the Head of the Department of Zoology, for providing the assistance in their research work.

Author details

Alpana Mukhuty[1*], Chandrani Fouzder[1], Snehasis Das[2] and Dipanjan Chattopadhyay[2]

1 Cell Signaling Laboratory, Department of Zoology, Visva-Bharati University, Santiniketan, India

2 Molecular Endocrinology Laboratory, Department of Zoology, Visva-Bharati University, Santiniketan, India

*Address all correspondence to: alpanamukhuty@yahoo.com

References

[1] Golson ML et al. High fat diet regulation of β-cell proliferation and β-cell mass. The Open Endocrinology Journal. 2010;**4**. DOI: 10.2174/1874216501004010066

[2] Weyer C et al. The natural history of insulin secretory dysfunction and insulin resistance in the pathogenesis of type 2 diabetes mellitus. The Journal of Clinical Investigation. 1999;**104**:787-794

[3] Cnop M et al. Progressive loss of b-cell function leads to worsening glucose tolerance in first-degree relatives of subjects with type 2 diabetes. Diabetes Care. 2007;**30**:677-682

[4] Brüning JC et al. Development of a novel polygenic model of NIDDM in mice heterozygous for IR and IRS-1 null alleles. Cell. 1997;**88**:561-572

[5] Meier JJ et al. β-cell replication is the primary mechanism subserving the postnatal expansion of β-cell mass in humans. Diabetes. 2008;**57**:1584-1594

[6] Butler AE et al. Adaptive changes in pancreatic β-cell fractional area and β-cell turnover in human pregnancy. Diabetologia. 2010;**53**:2167-2176

[7] Butler AE et al. Beta-cell deficit and increased beta-cell apoptosis in humans with type 2 diabetes. Diabetes. 2003;**52**:102-110

[8] Sachdeva MM et al. Minireview: Meeting the demand for insulin: Molecular mechanisms of adaptive postnatal beta-cell mass expansion. Molecular Endocrinology. 2009;**23**(6):747-758

[9] Fu Z et al. Regulation of insulin synthesis and secretion and pancreatic beta-cell dysfunction in diabetes. Current Diabetes Reviews. 2013;**9**(1):25-53

[10] Abel JJ. Crystalline insulin. Proceedings of the National Academy of Sciences. 1926;**12**:132-136

[11] Pittman I et al. Insulin biosynthesis, secretion, structure, and structure-activity relationships. 2004. Available from: http://diabetesmanager.pbworks.com/w/page/17680216/Insulin%20Biosynthesis,%20Secretion,%20Structure,%20and%20Structure-Activity%20Relationships

[12] Baker EN et al. The structure of 2 Zn pig insulin crystals at 1.5 a resolution. Philosophical Transactions. Royal Society of London. 1988;**B319**:369-456

[13] Blundell TL et al. The crystal structure of rhombohedral 2 zinc insulin. Cold Spring Harbor Symposia on Quantitative Biology. 1972;**36**:233-241

[14] Pullen RA et al. Receptor-binding region of insulin. Nature. 1976;**259**(5542):369-373

[15] Wollmer A et al. Phenol-promoted structural transformation of insulin in solution. Biological Chemistry Hoppe-Seyler. 1987;**368**(8):903-911

[16] Blundell TL et al. Three-dimensional atomic structure of insulin and its relationship to activity. Diabetes. 1972;**21**(2 Suppl):492-505

[17] Ogawa H et al. Effect of N-methylation of selected peptide bonds on the biological activity of insulin. [2-N-methylisoleucine-A] insulin and [3-N-methylvaline-A] insulin. International Journal of Peptide and Protein Research. 1987;**30**(4):460-473

[18] Schwartz G et al. Synthesis of des(tetrapeptide B(1-4)) and des(pentapeptide B(1-5)) human insulins. Two biologically

active analogues. Biochemistry. 1978;**17**(21):4550-4556

[19] Nakagawa SH et al. Implications of invariant residue LeuB6 in insulin-receptor interactions. The Journal of Biological Chemistry. 1991;**266**(18):11502-11509

[20] Chan SJ et al. A mutation in the B chain coding region is associated with impaired proinsulin conversion in a family with hyperproinsulinemia. Proceedings of the National Academy of Sciences of the United States of America. 1987;**84**(8):2194-2197

[21] Gruppuso PA et al. Familial hyperproinsulinemia due to a proposed defect in conversion of proinsulin to insulin. The New England Journal of Medicine. 1984;**311**(10):629-634

[22] Schwartz GP et al. A superactive insulin: [B10-aspartic acid] insulin(human). Proceedings of the National Academy of Sciences of the United States of America. 1987;**84**(18):6408-6411

[23] Suckale J et al. Pancreas islets in metabolic signaling—Focus on the beta-cell. Frontiers in Bioscience. 2008;**13**:7156-7171

[24] Chang TW et al. The metabolic fates of amino acids and the formation of glutamine in skeletal muscle. The Journal of Biological Chemistry. 1978;**253**(10):3685-3693

[25] Maechler P et al. Mitochondrial glutamate acts as a messenger in glucose-induced insulin exocytosis. Nature. 1999;**402**(6762):685-689

[26] Eto K et al. Role of NADH shuttle system in glucose-induced activation of mitochondrial metabolism and insulin secretion. Science. 1999;**283**(5404):981-985

[27] Bender K et al. The importance of redox shuttles to pancreatic beta-cell energy metabolism and function. Biochemical Society Transactions. 2006;**34**(Pt 5):811-814

[28] Mathilde D et al. Glucotoxicity inhibits late steps of insulin exocytosis. Endocrinology. 2007;**148**(4):1605-1614

[29] Crespin SR et al. Stimulation of insulin secretion by infusion of free fatty acids. The Journal of Clinical Investigation. 1969;**48**(10):1934-1943

[30] Roduit R et al. A role for the malonyl-CoA/long-chain acyl-CoA pathway of lipid signaling in the regulation of insulin secretion in response to both fuel and nonfuel stimuli. Diabetes. 2004;**53**(4):1007-1019

[31] Stein DT et al. Essentiality of circulating fatty acids for glucose-stimulated insulin secretion in the fasted rat. The Journal of Clinical Investigation. 1996;**97**(12):2728-2735

[32] Briscoe CP et al. The orphan G protein-coupled receptor GPR40 is activated by medium and long chain fatty acids. The Journal of Biological Chemistry. 2003;**278**(13):11303-11311

[33] Itoh Y et al. Free fatty acids regulate insulin secretion from pancreatic beta cells through GPR40. Nature. 2003;**422**(6928):173-176

[34] Prentki M. New insights into pancreatic beta-cell metabolic signaling in insulin secretion. European Journal of Endocrinology. 1996;**134**(3):272-286

[35] Prentki M et al. Ca^{2+}, cAMP, and phospholipid-derived messengers in coupling mechanisms of insulin secretion. Physiological Reviews. 1987;**67**(4):1185-1248

[36] Guenther B et al. Effects of a 48-h fat infusion on insulin secretion

and glucose utilization. Diabetes. 1995;**44**(10):1239-1242

[37] Sener A et al. L-leucine and a nonmetabolized analogue activate pancreatic islet glutamate dehydrogenase. Nature. 1980;**288**(5787):187-189

[38] Dixon G et al. A comparative study of amino acid consumption by rat islet cells and the clonal beta-cell line BRIN-BD11—The functional significance of L-alanine. The Journal of Endocrinology. 2003;**179**(3):447-454

[39] Tang CM et al. Glucagon-like peptide 2, a neurotransmitter with a newly discovered role in the regulation of food ingestion. Ugeskrift for Laeger. 2001;**163**(3):287-291

[40] MacDonald PE et al. The multiple actions of GLP-1 on the process of glucose-stimulated insulin secretion. Diabetes. 2002;**51**(Suppl 3):S434-S442

[41] MacDonald PE et al. Glucagon-like peptide-1 receptor activation antagonizes voltage-dependent repolarizing K(+) currents in beta-cells: A possible glucose-dependent insulinotropic mechanism. Diabetes. 2002;**51**(Suppl 3):S443-S447

[42] Orskov C. Glucagon-like peptide-1, a new hormone of the entero-insular axis. Diabetologia. 1992;**35**(8):701-711

[43] Flint A et al. Glucagon-like peptide 1 promotes satiety and suppresses energy intake in humans. The Journal of Clinical Investigation. 1998;**101**(3):515-520

[44] Nauck MA et al. Additive insulinotropic effects of exogenous synthetic human gastric inhibitory polypeptide and glucagon-like peptide-1-(7-36) amide infused at near-physiological insulinotropic hormone and glucose concentrations. The Journal of Clinical Endocrinology and Metabolism. 1993;**76**(4):912-917

[45] Ahren B. Islet G protein-coupled receptors as potential targets for treatment of type 2 diabetes. Nature Reviews. Drug Discovery. 2009;**8**(5):369-385

[46] Doyle ME, Egan JM. Mechanisms of action of glucagon-like peptide 1 in the pancreas. Pharmacology & Therapeutics. 2007;**113**(3):546-593

[47] Zhang Y et al. Positional cloning of the mouse obese gene and its human homologue. Nature. 1994;**372**(6505):425-432

[48] Rossetti L et al. Short term effects of leptin on hepatic gluconeogenesis and in vivo insulin action. The Journal of Biological Chemistry. 1997;**272**(44):27758-27763

[49] Montague CT et al. Congenital leptin deficiency is associated with severe early-onset obesity in humans. Nature. 1997;**387**(6636):903-908

[50] Fehmann HC et al. Leptin: A potent inhibitor of insulin secretion. Peptides. 1997;**18**(8):1267-1273

[51] Kulkarni RN et al. Leptin rapidly suppresses insulin release from insulinoma cells, rat and human islets and, in vivo, in mice. The Journal of Clinical Investigation. 1997;**100**(11):2729-2736

[52] Fehmann HC et al. Interaction of GLP-I and leptin at rat pancreatic B-cells: Effects on insulin secretion and signal transduction. Hormone and Metabolic Research. 1997;**29**(11):572-576

[53] Fehmann HC et al. Leptin inhibition of insulin secretion from isolated human islets. Acta Diabetologica. 1997;**34**(4):249-252

[54] Lupi R et al. Effects of acute or prolonged exposure to human leptin on isolated human islet function. Biochemical and Biophysical Research Communications. 1999;**256**(3):637-641

[55] Ahren B, Havel PJ. Leptin inhibits insulin secretion induced by cellular cAMP in a pancreatic B cell line (INS-1 cells). The American Journal of Physiology. 1999;**277**(4 Pt 2):R959-R966

[56] Poitout V et al. Inhibition of insulin secretion by leptin in normal rodent islets of Langerhans. Endocrinology. 1998;**139**(3):822-826

[57] Deroo BJ, Korach KS. Estrogen receptors and human disease. The Journal of Clinical Investigation. 2006;**116**(3):561-570

[58] Nadal A et al. Nongenomic actions of estrogens and xenoestrogens by binding at a plasma membrane receptor unrelated to estrogen receptor alpha and estrogen receptor beta. Proceedings of the National Academy of Sciences of the United States of America. 2000;**97**(21):11603-11608

[59] Sutter-Dub MT. Rapid non-genomic and genomic responses to progestogens, estrogens, and glucocorticoids in the endocrine pancreatic B cell, the adipocyte and other cell types. Steroids. 2002;**67**(2):77-93

[60] Nadal A et al. Rapid insulinotropic effect of 17beta-estradiol via a plasma membrane receptor. The FASEB Journal. 1998;**12**(13):1341-1348

[61] Stevenson JC et al. Hormone replacement therapy and the cardiovascular system. Nonlipid effects. Drugs. 1994;**47**(Suppl 2):35-41

[62] Brussaard HE et al. Short-term oestrogen replacement therapy improves insulin resistance, lipids and fibrinolysis in postmenopausal women with NIDDM. Diabetologia. 1997;**40**(7):843-849

[63] Ropero AB et al. A nonclassical estrogen membrane receptor triggers rapid differential actions in the endocrine pancreas. Molecular Endocrinology. 2002;**16**(3):497-505

[64] Hawkins MB et al. Identification of a third distinct estrogen receptor and reclassification of estrogen receptors in teleosts. Proceedings of the National Academy of Sciences of the United States of America. 2000;**97**(20):10751-10756

[65] Arendt J. Melatonin and the Mammalian Pineal Gland. London: Chapman and Hall; 1994

[66] Peschke E et al. Receptor (MT(1)) mediated influence of melatonin on cAMP concentration and insulin secretion of rat insulinoma cells INS-1. Journal of Pineal Research. 2002;**33**(2):63-71

[67] Kemp DM et al. Identification and functional characterization of melatonin Mel 1a receptors in pancreatic beta cells: Potential role in incretin-mediated cell function by sensitization of cAMP signaling. Molecular and Cellular Endocrinology. 2002;**191**(2):157-166

[68] Ramracheya RD et al. Function and expression of melatonin receptors on human pancreatic islets. Journal of Pineal Research. 2008;**44**(3):273-279

[69] Peschke E, Bach AG, Muhlbauer E. Parallel signaling pathways of melatonin in the pancreatic beta-cell. Journal of Pineal Research. 2006;**40**(2):184-191

[70] Peschke E. Melatonin, endocrine pancreas and diabetes. Journal of Pineal Research. 2008;**44**(1):26-40

[71] Bailey CJ et al. Melatonin inhibition of insulin secretion in the rat and mouse. Hormone Research. 1974;**5**(1):21-28

[72] Frankel BJ, Strandberg MJ. Insulin release from isolated mouse islets in vitro: No effect of physiological levels of melatonin or arginine vasotocin. Journal of Pineal Research. 1991;**11**(3-4):145-148

[73] Lyssenko V et al. Common variant in MTNR1B associated with increased risk of type 2 diabetes and impaired early insulin secretion. Nature Genetics. 2009;**41**(1):82-88

[74] Peschke E et al. Influence of melatonin and serotonin on glucose-stimulated insulin release from perifused rat pancreatic islets in vitro. Journal of Pineal Research. 1997;**23**(3):156-163

[75] Nishida S et al. Long-term melatonin administration reduces hyperinsulinemia and improves the altered fatty-acid compositions in type 2 diabetic rats via the restoration of Delta-5 desaturase activity. Journal of Pineal Research. 2002;**32**(1):26-33

[76] von Gall C et al. Mammalian melatonin receptors: Molecular biology and signal transduction. Cell and Tissue Research. 2002;**309**(1):151-162

[77] Bach AG et al. Melatonin stimulates inositol-1,4,5-trisphosphate and Ca^{2+} release from INS1 insulinoma cells. Journal of Pineal Research. 2005;**39**(3):316-323

[78] Godson C, Reppert SM. The Mel1a melatonin receptor is coupled to parallel signal transduction pathways. Endocrinology. 1997;**138**(1):397-404

[79] Sonksen PH. Insulin, growth hormone and sport. The Journal of Endocrinology. 2001;**170**(1):13-25

[80] Siddle K et al. Specificity in ligand binding and intracellular signalling by insulin and insulin-like growth factor receptors. Biochemical Society Transactions. 2001;**29**:513-525

[81] Guler HP et al. Effects of recombinant insulin-like growth factor I on insulin secretion and renal function in normal human subjects. Proceedings of the National Academy of Sciences of the United States of America. 1989;**86**(8):2868-2872

[82] Van Schravendijk CF et al. Direct effect of insulin and insulin-like growth factor-I on the secretory activity of rat pancreatic beta cells. Diabetologia. 1990;**33**(11):649-653

[83] Zhang F et al. Attenuation of insulin secretion by insulin-like growth factor binding protein-1 in pancreatic beta-cells. Biochemical and Biophysical Research Communications. 2007;**362**(1):152-157

[84] Malaisse W et al. Effects of adrenergic and cholinergic agents upon insulin Secretion in vitro. Endocrinology. 1967;**80**(5):975-978

[85] Vetterli L, Maechler P. Resveratrol-activated SIRT1 in liver and pancreatic β-cells: A Janus head looking to the same direction of metabolic homeostasis. Aging (Albany NY). 2011;**3**(4):444-449

[86] Maechler P et al. Role of mitochondria in beta-cell function and dysfunction. Advances in Experimental Medicine and Biology. 2010;**654**:193-216

[87] Moynihan KA et al. Increased dosage of mammalian Sir2 in pancreatic beta cells enhances glucose-stimulated insulin secretion in mice. Cell Metabolism. 2005;**2**:105-117

[88] Bordone L et al. Sirt1 regulates insulin secretion by repressing UCP2 in pancreatic beta cells. PLoS Biology. 2006;**4**:e31

[89] Kitamura YI et al. FoxO1 protects against pancreatic beta cell failure through NeuroD and MafA induction. Cell Metabolism. 2005;**2**:153-163

[90] Harbeck MC et al. Expression of insulin receptor mRNA and insulin receptor substrate 1 in pancreatic islet beta-cells. Diabetes. 1996;**45**:711-717

[91] Hennige AM et al. Overexpression of kinase-negative protein kinase Cdelta in pancreatic beta-cells protects mice from diet-induced glucose intolerance and beta-cell dysfunction. Diabetes. 2010;**59**:119-127

[92] Vetterli L et al. Resveratrol potentiates glucose-stimulated insulin secretion in INS-1E beta-cells and human islets through Sirt1 dependent mechanism. The Journal of Biological Chemistry. 2010;**286**:6049-6060

[93] Baur JA et al. Resveratrol improves health and survival of mice on a high-calorie diet. Nature. 2006;**444**:337-342

[94] Lagouge M et al. Resveratrol improves mitochondrial function and protects against metabolic disease by activating SIRT1 and PGC-1alpha. Cell. 2006;**127**:1109-1122

[95] Milne JC et al. Small molecule activators of SIRT1 as therapeutics for the treatment of type 2 diabetes. Nature. 2007;**450**:712-716

[96] Pfluger PT et al. Sirt1 protects against high-fat diet-induced metabolic damage. Proceedings of the National Academy of Sciences of the United States of America. 2008;**105**:9793-9798

[97] Banks AS et al. SirT1 gain of function increases energy efficiency and prevents diabetes in mice. Cell Metabolism. 2008;**8**:333-341

[98] Ling W et al. Activation of SIRT1 protects pancreatic β-cells against palmitate-induced dysfunction. Biochimica et Biophysica Acta. 2012;**1822**:1815-1825

[99] Gupta D et al. The role of peroxisome proliferator-activated receptor γ in pancreatic β-cell function and survival: Therapeutic implications for the treatment of type 2 diabetes mellitus. Diabetes, Obesity & Metabolism. 2010;**12**(12):1036-1047

[100] Yki-Jarvinen H. Thiazolidinediones. The New England Journal of Medicine. 2004;**351**:1106-1118

[101] Matsui J et al. Pioglitazone reduces islet triglyceride content and restores impaired glucose-stimulated insulin secretion in heterozygous peroxisome proliferator-activated receptor-gamma deficient mice on a high-fat diet. Diabetes. 2004;**53**:2844-2854

[102] Rosen ED et al. Targeted elimination of peroxisome proliferator-activated receptor gamma in beta cells leads to abnormalities in islet mass without compromising glucose homeostasis. Molecular and Cellular Biology. 2003;**23**:7222-7229

[103] Gupta D et al. In vivo and in vitro studies of a functional peroxisome proliferator-activated receptor gamma response element in the mouse pdx-1 promoter. The Journal of Biological Chemistry. 2008;**283**:32462-32470

[104] Chuang JC et al. Research resource: Nuclear hormone receptor expression in the endocrine pancreas. Molecular Endocrinology. 2008;**22**:2353-2363

[105] Moibi JA et al. Peroxisome proliferator activated receptor-{gamma} regulates expression of PDX-1 and NKX6. 1 in INS-1 cells. Diabetes. 2007;**56**:88-95

[106] Im SS et al. Identification and characterization of peroxisome proliferator response element in the mouse GLUT2 promoter. Experimental & Molecular Medicine. 2005;**37**:101-110

[107] Kim HI et al. Identification and functional characterization of the

peroxisomal proliferator response element in rat GLUT2 promoter. Diabetes. 2000;**49**:1517-1524

[108] Evans-Molina C et al. PPAR-{gamma} activation restores islet function in diabetic mice through reduction of ER stress and maintenance of euchromatin structure. Molecular and Cellular Biology. 2009;**29**:2053-2067

[109] Laybutt DR et al. Influence of diabetes on the loss of beta cell differentiation after islet transplantation in rats. Diabetologia. 2007;**50**:2117-2125

[110] Hull RL et al. Amyloid formation in human IAPP transgenic mouse islets and pancreas, and human pancreas, is not associated with endoplasmic reticulum stress. Diabetologia. 2009;**52**:1102-1111

[111] Brunham LR et al. Beta-cell ABCA1 influences insulin secretion, glucose homeostasis and response to thiazolidinedione treatment. Nature Medicine. 2007;**13**:340-347

[112] Vandewalle B et al. PPARgamma-dependent and -independent effects of rosiglitazone on lipotoxic human pancreatic islets. Biochemical and Biophysical Research Communications. 2008;**366**:1096-1101

[113] Lupi R et al. Rosiglitazone prevents the impairment of human islet function induced by fatty acids: Evidence for a role of PPARgamma2 in the modulation of insulin secretion. American Journal of Physiology. Endocrinology and Metabolism. 2004;**286**:E560-E567

[114] Maggi LBJ et al. Anti-inflammatory actions of 1 5-deoxy-delta 12, 14-prostaglandin J2 and troglitazone: Evidence for heat shock-dependent and -independent inhibition of cytokine-induced inducible nitric oxide synthase expression. Diabetes. 2000;**49**:346-355

[115] Kulkarni RN et al. Tissue-specific knockout of the insulin receptor in pancreatic beta cells creates an insulin secretory defect similar to that in type 2 diabetes. Cell. 1999;**96**:329-339

[116] Kim EK et al. Activation of peroxisome proliferator-activated receptor-γ protects pancreatic β-cells from cytokine-induced cytotoxicity via NFκB pathway. The International Journal of Biochemistry & Cell Biology. 2007;**39**:1260-1275

[117] Kim HS et al. PPAR-γ activation increases insulin secretion through the up-regulation of the free fatty acid receptor GPR40 in pancreatic β-cells. PLoS One. 2013;**8**(1):e50128

[118] Rulifson IC et al. Wnt signaling regulates pancreatic beta cell proliferation. Proceedings of the National Academy of Sciences of the United States of America. 2007;**104**(15):6247-6252

[119] Grant SF et al. Variant of transcription factor 7-like 2 (TCF7L2) gene confers risk of type 2 diabetes. Nature Genetics. 2006;**38**:320-323

[120] Ip W et al. The involvement of the wnt signaling pathway and TCF7L2 in diabetes mellitus: The current understanding, dispute, and perspective. Cell & Bioscience. 2012;**2**(1):28

[121] Lyssenko V et al. Mechanisms by which common variants in the TCF7L2 gene increase risk of type 2 diabetes. The Journal of Clinical Investigation. 2007;**117**:2155-2163

[122] Shu L et al. Transcription factor 7-like 2 regulates beta-cell survival and function in human pancreatic islets. Diabetes. 2008;**57**:645-653

[123] Elghazi L et al. Role of nutrients and mTOR signaling in the regulation of pancreatic progenitors development. Molecular Metabolism. 2017;**6**(6):560-573

[124] Gleason CE et al. The role of AMPK and mTOR in nutrient sensing in pancreatic beta-cells. The Journal of Biological Chemistry. 2007;**282**:10341-11035

[125] Fraenkel M et al. mTOR inhibition by rapamycin prevents β-cell adaptation to hyperglycemia and exacerbates the metabolic state in type 2 diabetes. Diabetes. 2008;**57**(4):945-957

[126] Um SH et al. Absence of S6K1 protects against age- and diet-induced obesity while enhancing insulin sensitivity. Nature. 2004;**431**:200-205

[127] Khamzina L et al. Increased activation of the mammalian target of rapamycin pathway in liver and skeletal muscle of obese rats: Possible involvement in obesity-linked insulin resistance. Endocrinology. 2005;**146**:1473-1481

[128] Shigeyama Y et al. Biphasic response of pancreatic beta-cell mass to ablation of tuberous sclerosis complex 2 in mice. Molecular and Cellular Biology. 2008;**28**:2971-2979

[129] Elghazi L et al. Decreased IRS signaling impairs beta-cell cycle progression and survival in transgenic mice overexpressing S6K in betacells. Diabetes. 2010;**59**:2390-2399

[130] Lorenzo P et al. Human pancreatic islets produce and secrete MCP-1/CCL2: Relevance in human islet transplantation. Diabetes. 2002;**51**(1):55-65

[131] Kutlu B et al. Molecular regulation of monocyte chemoattractant protein-1 expression in pancreatic β-cells. Diabetes. 2003;**52**(2):348-355

[132] Cai K et al. MCP-1 upregulates amylin expression in murine pancreatic β-cells through ERK/JNK-AP1 and NF-κB related signaling pathways independent of CCR2. PLoS One. 2011;**6**(5):e19559

[133] Yagishita Y et al. Nrf2 protects pancreatic β-cells from oxidative and nitrosative stress in diabetic model mice. Diabetes. 2014;**63**(2):605-618

[134] Fernandez-Millan E et al. Glucagon-like peptide-1 improves beta-cell antioxidant capacity via extracellular regulated kinases pathway and Nrf2 translocation. Free Radical Biology & Medicine. 2016;**95**:16-26

[135] Sato Y et al. Palmitate induces reactive oxygen species production and β-cell dysfunction by activating nicotinamide adenine dinucleotide phosphate oxidase through Src signaling. Journal of Diabetes Investigation. 2013;**5**(1):19-26

[136] Miettinen P et al. EGF receptor in pancreatic β-cell mass regulation. Biochemical Society Transactions. 2008;**36**(3):280-285

[137] Zarrouki B et al. Epidermal growth factor receptor signaling promotes pancreatic β-cell proliferation in response to nutrient excess in rats through mTOR and FOXM1. Diabetes. 2014;**63**(3):982-993

[138] Fonseca SG et al. Endoplasmic reticulum stress and pancreatic β-cell death. Trends in Endocrinology and Metabolism. 2011;**22**(7):266-274

[139] Lipson KL. Regulation of insulin biosynthesis in pancreatic beta cells by an endoplasmic reticulum-resident protein kinase IRE1. Cell Metabolism. 2006;**4**:245-254

[140] Lipson KL et al. The role of IRE1alpha in the degradation of insulin mRNA in pancreatic betaCells. PLoS One. 2008;**3**:e1648

[141] Hou ZQ et al. Involvement of chronic stresses in rat islet and INS-1 cell glucotoxicity induced by intermittent high glucose. Molecular and Cellular Endocrinology. 2008;**291**:71-78

[142] Jonas JC et al. Glucose regulation of islet stress responses and beta-cell failure in type 2 diabetes. Diabetes, Obesity & Metabolism. 2009;**11**(Suppl 4):65-81

[143] Cnop M et al. Selective inhibition of eukaryotic translation initiation factor 2 alpha dephosphorylation potentiates fatty acid-induced endoplasmic reticulum stress and causes pancreatic beta-cell dysfunction and apoptosis. The Journal of Biological Chemistry. 2007;**282**:3989-3997

[144] Karaskov E et al. Chronic palmitate but not oleate exposure induces endoplasmic reticulum stress, which may contribute to INS-1 pancreatic beta-cell apoptosis. Endocrinology. 2006;**147**:3398-3407

[145] Kharroubi I et al. Free fatty acids and cytokines induce pancreatic beta-cell apoptosis by different mechanisms: Role of nuclear factor-kappaB and endoplasmic reticulum stress. Endocrinology. 2004;**145**:5087-5096

[146] Cardozo AK et al. Cytokines downregulate the sarcoendoplasmic reticulum pump Ca^{2+} ATPase 2b and deplete endoplasmic reticulum Ca^{2+}, leading to induction of endoplasmic reticulum stress in pancreatic beta-cells. Diabetes. 2005;**54**:452-461

[147] Wali JA et al. Activation of the NLRP3 inflammasome complex is not required for stress-induced death of pancreatic islets. PLoS One. 2014;**9**(11):e113128

[148] Jourdan T et al. Activation of the Nlrp3 inflammasome in infiltrating macrophages by endocannabinoids mediates beta cell loss in type 2 diabetes. Nature Medicine. 2013;**19**(9):1132-1140

[149] Zhou R et al. Thioredoxin-interacting protein links oxidative stress to inflammasome activation. Nature Immunology. 2010;**11**:136-141

[150] Garay-Malpartida HM et al. Toll-like receptor 4 (TLR4) expression in human and murine pancreatic beta-cells affects cell viability and insulin homeostasis. BMC Immunology. 2011;**12**:18

[151] Eguchi K et al. Saturated fatty acid and TLR signaling link β-cell dysfunction and islet inflammation. Cell Metabolism. 2012;**15**(4):518-533

[152] Li J et al. TLR4 is required for the obesity-induced pancreatic beta cell dysfunction. Acta Biochimica et Biophysica Sinica. 2013;**45**(12):1030-1038

[153] Shen X et al. Fetuin-a promoteslipotoxicity in β-cells through the TLR4 signaling pathway and the role of pioglitazone in anti-lipotoxicity. Molecular and Cellular Endocrinology. 2015;**412**:1-11

[154] Mukhuty A et al. Palmitate induced Fetuin-A secretion from pancreatic β-cells adversely affects its function and elicits inflammation. Biochemical and Biophysical Research Communications. 2017;**491**:1118-1124

[155] Amisten S et al. An atlas and functional analysis of G-prote n coupled receptors in human islets of Langerhans. Pharmacology & Therapeutics. 2013;**139**(3):359-391

[156] Mancini AD et al. The fatty acid receptor FFA1/GPR40 a decade later: How much do we know? Trends in Endocrinology and Metabolism. 2013;**24**(8):398-407

[157] Sassmann A et al. The Gq/G11-mediated signaling pathway is critical for autocrine potentiation of insulin secretion in mice. The Journal of Clinical Investigation. 2010;**120**(6):2184-2193

Chapter 2

Pathogenesis of Type 2 Diabetes Mellitus

Pilar Durruty, María Sanzana and Lilian Sanhueza

Abstract

Type 2 diabetes mellitus (DM2) results from the interaction between genetic and environmental factors which cause insulin resistance (IR) and deficit in insulin secretion. Genes encoding insulin-related enzymes or protein factors are candidates for the disease, most probably the insulin receptor substrate-1 (IRS-1), phosphoinositide 3-kinase (PI-3 K), calpain 10, and transcription factor 7-like 2 genes. Environmental factors that favor DM2 are android obesity, aging, glucotoxicity, and lipotoxicity. IR is the result of less insulin receptor binding, of less phosphorylation of the receptor, of IRS-1, of PI-3 K, and of glucose uptake by glucose transporters. At the hepatic level, glucose is produced by gluconeogenesis: in the muscle there is less glycogen deposition, and in adipocytes there is greater release of free fatty acids (FFA). Insulin secretion is the main pathogenic factor; relative insulin hyposecretion is not capable of compensating for the IR. Reduced incretin effect, hyperglucagonemia, and increased renal glucose reabsorption favor hyperglycemia. Disturbance of the microbiota releases proinflammatory adipocytokines which contribute to IR. Reactive oxygen species generation, caused by hyperglycemia and FFA, results in a decrease in insulin synthesis and action and also endoplasmic reticulum stress and mitochondrial dysfunction. Knowledge about the pathogenesis of DM2 has allowed the development of drugs for its treatment.

Keywords: type 2 diabetes, pathogenesis, environment, sleep disturbances, insulin resistance, glucotoxicity, lipotoxicity, microbiota

1. Introduction

Type 2 diabetes mellitus (DM2) is a complex metabolic and endocrine disorder resulting from the interaction between genetic and environmental factors, which cause different degrees of alteration in insulin functionality on peripheral tissues, as well as in the pancreatic β cell. Underlying pathologies such as excess weight and obesity, particularly of the android type, are the main factors that favor the development of DM2 [1, 2].

In absolute terms, insulinemia of diabetic subjects may be similar to those of euglycemic individuals but are proportionally insufficient in the hyperglycemia states. Reduced insulin action, for determined levels of the hormone, is known as insulin resistance (IR). When β cells undergo IR, initially there is insulin hypersecretion which compensates for the lack of hormonal action. Hyperglycemia only manifests when there exists a relative insulin hyposecretion to the glucose stimulus [3].

2. Natural history of DM2

DM2 is a progressive disease that develops in stages. Its natural history probably begins 10–20 years before its clinical onset, as a preclinical period with IR [4].

Hyperinsulinemia is initially capable of maintaining normal fasting and postprandial glycemias. This stage would be associated with increased levels of free fatty acids (FFA) in the obese IR patient.

Subsequently, and before DM2 manifests, IR is maintained, but the secretory capacity of the β cell begins to decline and glycemias rise, reaching abnormality levels for fasting glycemia and glucose intolerance, which are prediabetes stages. In these periods, chronic hyperglycemia is an important factor in the perpetuation of damage to the pancreatic β cells; as it increases and IR is maintained, glycemic levels progressively increase until finally clinical diabetes is established.

The stages of the pathogenesis of DM2 are shown in **Figure 1**.

The insulin secretory defects observed in DM2 contribute to IR. During the evolution of DM2, the IR state is maintained, and the insulin secretory capacity gradually decreases, arriving at an insulin hyposecretion in which it will be necessary, in some cases, to start insulin therapy.

Hyperglycemia in DM2 not only represents the biochemical manifestation of the disease, but it is rather, in itself, a permanent factor responsible for maintaining the diabetic state.

We will now refer to the multiple factors involved in the genesis of DM2.

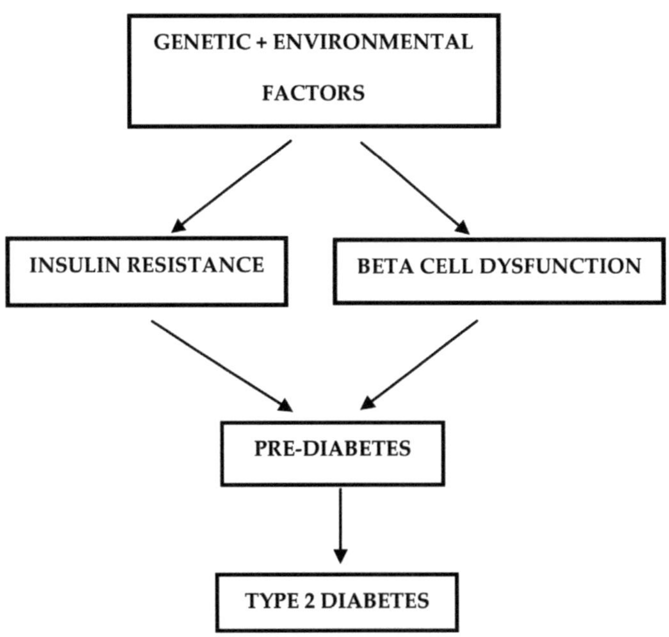

Figure 1.
Stages in pathogenesis of type 2 diabetes.

3. Genetic factors of DM2

Presently, DM2 is considered to be a disease with a strong hereditary component. Thus, 35–50% of the patients have diabetic relatives, a number that is lower (15%) in subjects not having this pathology. If a survey for DM2 is conducted on the patients' parents, 10–30% of them have the disease in comparison to 1–6% in healthy controls.

In the Framingham Offspring Study, it was found that if one of the parents was diabetic, in the offspring the relative risk was 3.6; if both parents had the disease, it rose to 6.0. This study indicates that the risk for diabetes in sons or daughters of diabetic parents is similar regardless if it is the father or the mother who has the disease [5]. In monozygotic twins, there is up to 96% match for DM2, a percentage that falls to less than 50% in fraternal twins.

All genes that encode enzymes or protein factors associated with insulin secretion and action are possible candidates for the disease. It has been published that the hereditary factor is stronger than the environmental factor for the secretory defect. In IR, genetic and environmental factors have 50% participation each.

Table 1 shows the most relevant candidate genes for DM2, which are related to the insulin secretion defect and to IR.

Each gene has been found to be altered in approximately 10% of the DM2 patients studied. Therefore, it is necessary for the individual to have at least 10 defective genes for the disease to develop. Besides, in the various populations, different genotypes involved would exist, and differences would appear also in individuals of a same ethnic group.

3.1 Genetic defects of IR

Genetic mutations have been found in certain protein factors and enzymes associated with the transmission of the insulin signal inside the effector cell, which would allow to partly explain the IR of DM2 [6–8]. In the insulin receptor substrate-1 (IRS-1) gene, the mutation of glycine to arginine at codon 972 is twice more prevalent in Caucasian DM2 patients than in nondiabetic controls.

Insulin resistance genes
1. Directly associated with lower glucose uptake • Insulin receptor substrate gene • Phosphoinositide 3-kinase gene 2. Explaining the obesity-type 2 diabetes relationship • β-3 adrenergic receptor gene • Tumor necrosis factor alpha gene • Peroxisome proliferator-activated receptor gene 3. Adipocytokines in obesity • Leptin gene • Resistin gene • Adiponectin gene 4. Lipid metabolism • Lipoprotein lipase gene • Fatty acid-binding protein gene 5. The thermogenesis obesity relationship • Uncoupling protein gene
Insulin secretion genes
• Insulin receptor substrate gene • Calpain 10 gene • K+ inwardly rectifier channel gene

Table 1.
Candidate genes of type 2 diabetes.

For phosphoinositide 3-kinase (PI-3 K), it has been demonstrated that in DM2 its synthesis is lower because the messenger RNA levels are lower.

In the relation of obesity with DM2, correlation, among the possible genes involved, mention is made of the tumor necrosis factor alpha (TNFα) gene, a polymorphism in its promoter consisting of the substitution of guanine to adenine at position 308, which originates higher TNFα synthesis in obese IR patients. The finding regarding leptin is very interesting, in studies on thousands of cases since only five have genetic mutations for the hormone, suggesting that obesity in DM2 humans would be associated with leptin resistance at the level of its receptors. On the other side, the adiponectin gene is located on chromosome 3q27, and in this position, a locus has been found which confers susceptibility to DM2. For resistin, it has been reported that its genetic expression is four times higher in abdominal adipose tissue than in subcutaneous adipose tissue.

The hereditary basis of IR in DM2 is extremely complex, moreover, when the obesity factor is included having its own polygenic component. DM2 patients have different degrees of IR with probably different genetic origins; this explains why their clinical behavior is singular.

3.2 Genetic defects in insulin secretion

In DM2, the genes encoding the different protein components that participate in the mechanism of insulin synthesis and secretion are potential candidates [9, 10]. Among the most likely ones is the IRS-2 gene, which is very interesting because a polymorphism has been described which predicts anomalies both in insulin secretion and action. In 2000, a false announcement was issued regarding the discovery of the gene of DM2, referring to the calpain 10 (CAPN10) gene that encodes a family of calpain enzymes, which are calcium-activated proteases that take part in the regulation of insulin exocytosis in β cells. It was published that in Pima Indians, a specific combination of CAPN10 alleles triplicated the risk of DM2. However, in recent years, the transcription factor 7-like 2 (TCF7L2) gene has appeared to be more relevant in the genetic susceptibility to DM2, since a polymorphism of this gene has been found in several ethnic groups of DM2 patients. This factor is associated to a reduced response to glucagon-like peptide-1 (GLP-1) because GLP-1 expression in enteroendocrine cells is regulated by TCF7L2, which would have as a final consequence, a failure in β cell proliferation and in insulin secretion; thus, variants of the TCF7L2 gene would contribute to the risk for DM2.

It can be said that DM2 is a polygenic disease with many susceptibility genes, each with a slight impact on its pathogenesis but giving origin to several subgroups of DM2 on account of their genetic differences. Thus, in the various individuals and in the different ethnic groups, genetic heterogeneity results in variable degrees of alterations both in insulin secretion and action.

4. Environmental factors of DM2

Environmental factors are considered to be all situations that favor the development of this type of diabetes.

4.1 Obesity

General obesity, and in particular the android type, is the main environmental factor in the genesis of DM2. In our experience, at diagnosis of DM2, 80% of the patients are obese.

Historically, it was believed that fat tissue was metabolically neutral, being only an energy reservoir. In recent years, it is considered to be a real endocrine organ with a huge importance in the pathogenesis of DM2 and IR [11].

The increase in visceral adipose tissue results in higher levels of FFA that activate the β isoform of protein kinase C (PKCβ) and inhibit glucose transport-4 (GLUT-4) translocation to the cell membrane, reducing glucose entry into insulin target tissues. TNFα and interleukin-6 (IL-6), by phosphorylating IRS-1 on serine/threonine residues and not on tyrosine, disrupt the correct transmission of the insulin signal.

Adipose tissue also secretes several hormones known as adipocytokines; among them we will refer, in relation to the increase in IR, to leptin, adiponectin, and resistin. DM2 patients exhibit elevated leptin levels, favoring obesity due to greater food intake and lower caloric expenditure. In humans, the defect is a resistance to leptin action at the hypothalamic receptor level, with obesity developing as these receptors become insensitive to leptin. Adiponectin is the only adipocytokine whose circulating levels are diminished in obesity. It is interesting to point out that the low adiponectin levels are observed particularly in coronary patients, constituting a risk marker for this pathology. In respect of resistin, there has been much controversy regarding its role in obesity and DM2. Its overexpression is associated to IR, dyslipidemia, and DM2, through inhibition of cell glucose uptake.

4.2 Aging

The influence of age on the development of DM2 is indisputable only by reviewing the universal epidemiology of this type of diabetes, which shows a progressive increment of its prevalence rates with increasing age. Glucose tolerance deteriorates with aging, which has been attributed to the loss of muscular mass and increase in adipose tissue (sarcopenia), especially in sedentary individuals, increasing IR in susceptible subjects [12].

It has been proposed that at an older age, mitochondrial functions decline favoring IR and, on the other side, leptin resistance rises intensifying visceral fat deposition, increasing IR and inducing DM2.

4.3 Psychological stress

Acute psychological stress has been acknowledged for many years as a factor which favors the onset of diabetes. This is because sympathetic activation reduces the functionality of the pancreatic β cell, diminishing insulin secretion.

At the same time, in the muscle there is a decline in insulin sensitivity, glucose uptake, and glycogen deposition, all of which elevates glycemia and clinically favors the development of DM2.

Among the psychosocial factors related to this type of diabetes, depression in its different degrees has been widely studied, and a bidirectional association has been found between both disorders. It is bidirectional in the sense that depression induces DM2 and diabetics suffer from 30% more depressive states than nondiabetics [13].

The Cardiovascular Health Study demonstrated, in elderly adults, that those who reported strong depressive symptoms developed DM2 more frequently than their non-depressive peers. This association cannot be totally explained by differences in the risk factors for DM2. It is likely that both disorders have a common feature [14].

Although the intimate mechanism of this association is not known, it has been speculated that it could be related to inflammation, considering that inflammatory markers are present in diabetes and in depressive states. Some authors have found elevated C-reactive protein levels in these cases, but this has not been confirmed by others.

It has been established that depressive subjects are physically less active and that, due to their psychic disorders, also have poor eating habits, both behaviors favoring obesity, IR, and DM2. Diabetics are highly sensitive to the effects of physical stress, which is related to adrenergic stimulation that could reduce insulin secretion and glucose utilization.

In recent years, abnormal glucose metabolism has been correlated with various sleep disturbances, such as duration, fragmentation, quality, respiratory function, obstructive sleep apnea, hypoxemia, and circadian rhythm. This situation is explained by an increase in cortisol, growth hormone, inflammatory markers, and adipocyte function. There also exists a reduction in brain glucose utilization, with an increase in ghrelin, a situation that leads to obesity. This is reflected in an increase in IR and a reduction in β cell function, ultimately favoring hyperglycemia and DM2 [15].

4.4 Glucotoxicity and lipotoxicity

The concepts of glucotoxicity and lipotoxicity, related to DM2, appear in the 1990s, supported by experimental studies in animals which have been subsequently confirmed in humans. At present, glucotoxicity is defined as the adverse effects produced by chronic hyperglycemia on cell structures and functions. Hyperglycemia would cause an inhibition of the hormone synthesis through a decrease in messenger RNA for insulin; therefore, glucose would be capable of inducing damage at the level of the genetic information which is indispensable for a correct insulin synthesis [16].

Other mechanisms involved in glucotoxicity would be the lower activity of phospholipase C, an enzyme necessary for the formation of inositide phosphates which participate in insulin secretion by increasing the intracellular calcium level. Cytotoxicity to the β cell by glucose, acting as a free radical, is also possible, causing greater β cell apoptosis.

In 1963, Randle proposed that the increase in FFA, as a result of the degradation of triglycerides, causes peripheral IR. A great FFA mobilization due to greater lipolysis induces an increase in FFA oxidation in the muscle and the liver, with less glucose utilization in the former and higher hepatic gluconeogenesis; this leads to hyperglycemia plus inhibition of insulin secretion, which further elevates serum glucose levels. FFA are deposited in the muscle as triglycerides, ectopic deposits which favor IR. In the β cells, reactive oxygen species (ROS) increase, thus reducing insulin gene expression and secretion [17]. Therefore, a dual mechanism is acknowledged to lipotoxicity in the pathogenesis of DM2: it favors IR and has a direct deleterious effect on β cells. Probably, ROS produce less insulin secretion due to a lower GLUT-2 activity.

Glucotoxicity and lipotoxicity, disclosed separately for didactic reasons, coparticipate in the genesis of DM2 and interact together causing structural and functional damage in β cells and in target organs. Thus, glucotoxicity describes more accurately the reality of the chronic deleterious process. Glucolipotoxicity is capable of causing inflammation in pancreatic β cells and in the peripheral tissues where insulin acts. In the β cells, an activation of the nuclear factor kappa beta (NF-kβ) pathway occurs, increasing the production of NF-kβ which is an inflammatory cytokine. In the visceral adipose tissue, there is a decrease in adiponectin which is anti-inflammatory (insulin-sensitizing) and an increase in the proinflammatory cytokines: leptin, TNFα, and IL-6.

This chronic low-grade inflammatory state is referred to as a metainflammation [18].

4.5 Oxidative stress

ROS, generated both by hyperglycemia and increased FFA levels, would have the most important role in the onset and progression of DM2. In β cells, ROS [18] cause a decrease in insulin synthesis and secretion; since β cells have a low antioxidant capacity, excessive ROS production results in an imbalance of the redox state, tilting the balance toward oxidation. In peripheral tissues that are targets for insulin, ROS favor inactivation of insulin signal transmission. It has also been observed that inflammation, mainly through the increase in IL-6 and TNFα, favors IR and β cell dysfunction.

On the other side, the production of chemicals used worldwide in different activities including the food industry, probably through ROS generation, has increased progressively since 1940. In the USA, a direct relationship has been found between the production curves of synthetic organic chemicals and the prevalence of diabetes and other pathologies [19]. The Environmental Protection Agency has defined as endocrine-disrupting chemicals, exogenous agents that interfere with the production, secretion, transport, metabolism, binding, action, or clearance of hormones.

4.6 Endoplasmic reticulum stress and endothelial dysfunction

The endoplasmic reticulum actively participates in protein synthesis, producing the correct folding of proteins by means of chaperones, which are helpers of this process. Activating signals such as hyperglycemia increase the demand for insulin synthesis, causing endoplasmic reticulum stress in β cells; this induces apoptotic pathways as a normal adaptive metabolic response to a metabolic load. In DM2, the endoplasmic reticulum stress caused by glucotoxicity and inflammatory cytokines can lead to β cell dysfunction and death [20].

The β cell mitochondrion participates in insulin synthesis and in exocytosis. In diabetes, a mitochondrial dysfunction occurs: the mitochondrial membrane proteins are diminished, and transcriptional changes occur in their formation. Mitochondrial dysfunction, induced by glucotoxicity, results in β cell failure, increase in ROS, and oxidative stress.

In IR, the excess of circulating fatty acids associated with the reduction in the number of mitochondria causes an increment in the level of intracellular FFA and also of diacylglycerol. These molecules activate PKC which in turn activates the serine kinase cascade, leading to an increment in the phosphorylation of the serine residues in IRS-1 and preventing the phosphorylation of tyrosine residues, which in turn inhibits PI-3 K activity, finally resulting in the suppression of insulin-induced glucose transport [21].

4.7 Diet and nutrients

In recent years, a special interest has aroused for studying the influence of the diet in general and of different nutrients in particular, on the development of DM2.

There is a consensus in that a healthy diet with no caloric excess and a suitable physical activity are the most effective measures for preventing DM2. There is also clinical and biological evidence that excessive sugar consumption promotes the development of DM2 and of cardiovascular disease [22].

The effect of dietary fat on the risk for DM2 is not absolutely clarified, and some studies have even provided contradictory results; but there exists a consensus in that the quality of the fat is more important than the total amount. Dietary fat is not only a source of energy, but also fatty acids affect cell metabolism. Monounsaturated fatty acids and trans-fatty acids would not be associated with a higher incidence of DM2.

In relation to dietary fats, arrives at more categorical conclusions indicating that a diet high in monounsaturated fatty acids (olive oil) and polyunsaturated fatty acids of marine origin is associated with low risk of DM2 [23]. This is confirmed by the fact that consumption of Mediterranean diet, high in monounsaturated fatty acids from vegetable oils and polyunsaturated fatty acids from fish, reduces the risk for DM2.

For a long time, it was believed that free consumption of fructose had no negative effects on the body, since it does not require insulin for its metabolism. Recent studies demonstrate the exact opposite, stating that excessive intake favors metabolic syndrome. In recent years, the high fructose consumption in corn syrups in the USA is correlated with the increased prevalence of DM2, obesity, and cardiovascular disease.

The so-called fructose hypothesis postulates that a high fructose content in the diet induces activation of peroxisome proliferator-activated receptor gamma (PPAR-ϒ) responsible for IR, lipogenesis, and DM2 [24]. Besides, the fructose load with the resulting hepatic stress causes the release of proinflammatory cytokines such as TNFα that induces IR and favors the development of DM2.

The association between gluten intake and DM2 has been the subject matter of recent studies. In US healthy men and women, an inverse correlation has been found between gluten intake and incidence of DM2.

Subjects receiving a diet with high gluten content, followed up for 20–28 years, exhibit low DM2 rates [25]. The cause would be in that subjects who eat gluten-rich foods also receive an elevated supply of cereal fiber. The mechanism through which gluten reduces the risk of DM2 is unknown but is probably related to favorable changes in gut microbiota.

Presently, the effect of vitamin D supplements at pharmacological dosages in the prevention of both type 1 and type 2 diabetes is being debated. Epidemiologic studies demonstrate a relationship between vitamin D deficiency and DM2, as well as the higher frequency of this type of diabetes in areas with low sun exposure. In prospective studies of up to 20 years in humans, it has been demonstrated that the incidence of DM2 decreases by providing a daily supplement of 800 IU of vitamin D [26]. However, other studies do not show the same results; it could be concluded that supplying vitamin D to persons at risk for diabetes is an advisable measure, even though there is still not enough scientific evidence to support this position.

5. Deficit in insulin secretion

In DM2 patients, deficit in insulin secretion is the building block of its pathogenesis. It has been found that the disturbances caused are both quantitative and qualitative and are present in variable degrees in the patients.

When the secretory disorder appears, hyperglycemia manifests. It has been demonstrated that, in general, individuals exhibiting the most severe hyposecretion have the highest glycemias. The graphic relationship of fasting and postprandial glycemias versus insulinemias is very well known and gives origin to the inverted U or Starling curve; at low glucose values, insulinemias are also low and then the relationship is inverse, and at higher glycemias, there are lower insulinemias [27].

In DM2 patients, the lack of insulin response to glucose worsens with the years of evolution of the disease and is accentuated with the persistent hyperglycemias (glucotoxicity). Once glycemia rises, a vicious circle is produced because glucose on its own causes changes in β cells, paradoxically slowing down insulin secretion [28].

DM2 patients exhibit changes in the biphasic insulin secretion curve under a stimulus of intravenous glucose; the first phase is lost, the second phase shows less elevation and is more prolonged in time than in the normal curve. These alterations, which are present since the prediabetes state, reduce the effectiveness of insulin. Besides, in DM2 patients, there are a lower number of pulses of insulin secretion under glucose stimulus [29]. Similar to other hormones, insulin is more effective when secreted in pulses that released continuously.

At the anatomical level, in the pancreas of DM2 patients, there is a 40% reduction of the β cell mass, which on its own does not explain the hyposecretion. In this respect, the theory of low birth weight, also called the theory of the thrifty gene or of feast and famine, is very attractive. In those patients, their reduced pancreas does not allow to compensate the insulin demand when they are obese, subsequently developing DM2 [30]. The reduction in β cell mass could be due to an increase in apoptosis and autophagy that would exceed the islet regenerative capacity.

In DM2, a morphological change that has been extensively studied is the amyloid deposition in the islets of Langerhans, a disturbance that may lead to accelerated death of β cells with the consequent decrease of insulin secretion. It has been reported that the presence of amyloid coincides with or precedes hyperglycemia, favoring β cell apoptosis [31].

Amyloid is constituted by a peptide initially named amylin and presently referred to as islet amyloid polypeptide (IAPP), normally produced by β cells. This amyloid forms fibrils that are cytotoxic to these cells through an oxidative stress mechanism; IAPP overexposure would favor DM2 development. It has not yet been clarified whether the excess of amyloid deposition is caused by the hyperglycemia or precedes the diagnosis of DM2.

At present, epigenetics is considered to be a factor of DM2 and other diseases; these are interactions between genes and environment that occur in individuals through small chemical modifications that are capable of regulating the expression of the DM2 genes especially related to insulin secretion [32].

6. Insulin resistance

IR, defined as a lower biological activity of the hormone in its different metabolic actions for a certain concentration, is the first abnormality detected in the evolution of DM2 and is already present in the prediabetes state.

IR plays a main role in DM2 development together with the insulin secretion defect, both disorders having genetic bases that have been extensively studied but not well defined to date, influenced by epigenetic factors that can act since intrauterine life.

IR, obesity, and DM2 are highly interrelated. In 95% of the cases, IR presents in subjects with excess weight or obesity will subsequently develop DM2. Although IR is present in almost all patients with DM2, the degrees of IR are very variable in different individuals; besides, a proportion of IR comes from obesity itself, and the other is characteristic of DM2.

IR is expressed in the liver, muscle, and adipose tissue with different intensities in the different individuals.

In DM2 due to IR, hyperglycemia occurs through three mechanisms: excessive hepatic production of glucose (gluconeogenesis), decrease in its uptake by peripheral tissues (muscle and adipose tissue), and increase in FFA resulting from a greater lipolysis in the adipocytes. FFA competes with glucose as a source of energy contributing to increase glycemia and inhibit glucose entry through the cell membrane [3].

6.1 IR in the liver

A positive correlation has been demonstrated between fasting glucose and hepatic gluconeogenesis, such that as the latter descends, basal glycemia levels also descend. Therefore, the hepatic gluconeogenesis that produces glucose in an environment of elevated glycemia levels is abnormal and of very important in maintaining fasting hyperglycemia in DM2 patients. The mechanism through which hepatic glucose production increases would be an elevated supply of FFA from adipose tissue, which through the metabolites of the Krebs cycle, serve as a substrate for gluconeogenesis. In the liver, at least two types of alterations have been found: the already mentioned increase in hepatic gluconeogenesis and an incapacity both of insulin and of glycemia to inhibit glucose production. In individuals with IR, the hepatic glucose cycle is increased due to a higher activity of glucose-6-phosphatase that dephosphorylates glucose-6-phosphate, which once dephosphorylated cannot be metabolized in the glycolysis such that glucose enters the circulation favoring hyperglycemia.

6.2 IR in the muscle

Glucose utilization by the skeletal muscle is mainly mediated by insulin and reaches about 5 g/hour in the postabsorptive state. In DM2 patients, this process is severely disrupted, glucose uptake is decreased, and the amount of stored glycogen is reduced.

Glycogenesis is approximately 60% lower due to a lower activity of the muscle glycogen synthase (GS) [33]. In the IR state, insulin is incapable of stimulating muscle GS; there is excess glucose in the postabsorptive state, but it is not deposited in the form of glycogen, such that this genetic defect directly contributes to post-prandial hyperglycemia.

6.3 IR in adipose tissue

In DM2 patients with IR and low insulin levels, a greater lipolysis occurs in the adipocytes increasing the concentration of circulating FFA, particularly during the night; the capacity of insulin, in these cases, is being insufficient to maintain the FFA plasma levels within the normal range.

FFA, as already mentioned, contribute to elevate fasting glycemia through gluconeogenesis, which would be the main defect, and additionally reduce glucose uptake and oxidation in the muscle.

Increased FFA inhibits the activity of pyruvate dehydrogenase, an enzyme that participates in the final stage of glycolysis, thus slowing down glucose degradation and energy production by glucose metabolism.

The higher supply of long-chain FFA by the fatty acid-binding protein-2 (FABP-2) for their oxidation as a source of energy is another mechanism of competition with glucose.

Regulation of FFA metabolism is highly sensitive to insulin levels and is probably one of the first actions that are lost when insulinemia decreases and the individual is IR.

The metabolic pathways of IR in the liver, muscle and adipose tissue of DM2 patients is seen in **Figure 2**.

6.4 Cellular mechanisms

In DM2 patients, IR is caused by alterations in the insulin receptor, and mainly postreceptor changes subsequent to insulin receptor binding. Disturbances at the receptor level would be caused by obesity of the patients and postreceptor ones would be more specific to DM2.

Normally, insulin action in relation to glucose uptake occurs by insulin binding to its receptor which is a tyrosine kinase that is activated by autophosphorylation on tyrosine, this being the first step. Subsequently, second messengers are produced, among others IRS and PI-3 K, which are also activated by phosphorylation on tyrosine; then, GLUT migrate from the intracellular space to the cell membrane to take up glucose from the blood stream through facilitated diffusion, which is a selective

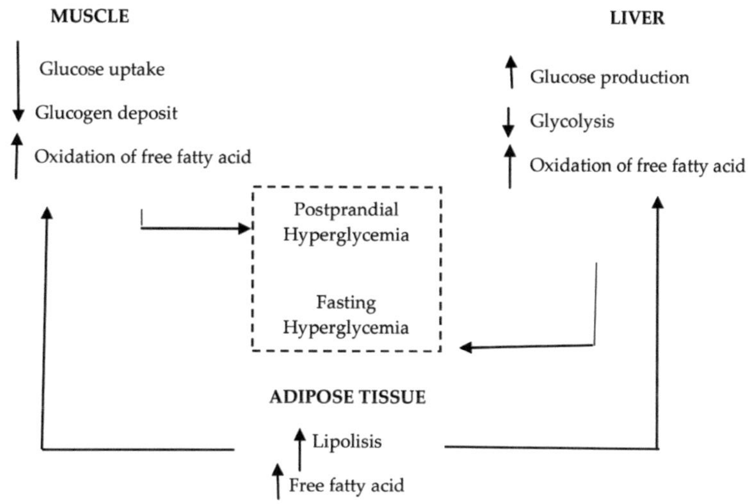

Figure 2.
Mechanism involved in insulin resistance in the liver, muscle and adipose tissue.

translocation of a molecule against its gradient by transporters. As a last stage for ending the signal transmission, the receptor is inactivated by a dephosphorylating mechanism, a process in which protein-tyrosine phosphatase-1B (PTP-1B) participates.

In DM2, part of the IR is caused by a reduction of insulin binding to its receptors; however, defects in the protein substrates and in the enzymes, inside the cells, would be of greater importance, and they correspond to postreceptor defects. The abnormalities of the receptor do not explain the great IR of DM2 patients; therefore, postreceptor defects are considered to contribute in higher proportion to cause this disturbance.

Numerous studies have demonstrated that insulin receptor binding in the various tissues of DM2 patients is decreased by 50% in obese subjects and by 20% in normal weight subjects. Besides, the autophosphorylation capacity of the receptor is 40% less than in nondiabetic individuals. The decrease in kinase activity of the receptor is a relatively specific damage of the diabetic state, which can be due to an intrinsic enzymatic defect of the receptor. In DM2, only a small fraction of the total receptors is capable of autophosphorylation under insulin stimulus; therefore, the activity of the receptors is reduced leading to lower action of the hormone, which is IR.

In DM2 patients, there could exist deterioration in insulin-mediated IRS-1 phosphorylation when a proportion of these protein factors that phosphorylate on serine (not on tyrosine) are inactivated. Consequently, the insulin signal transmission is lower inside the cell [34], and glucose transport is reduced due to diminished PI-3 K activity. There is also a significant reduction in the number of glucose transporters available in the cell membrane, which would be due to a disorder in their distribution as they remain within an inactive intracellular pool, the final result being hyperglycemia. Increased FFA reduces glucose transport translocation through inhibition of PKCβ activity and lower GLUT phosphorylation.

The β cell is in charge of responding to these higher demands caused by IR, increasing insulin synthesis in order to preserve normal levels of fasting and postprandial glycemias. In DM2, insulin is incapable of responding to the demands of IR; it is evident that the ability of the β cell for secreting insulin under the glucose stimulus for maintaining glycemic homeostasis is lost in DM2.

DM2 does not develop if there is no β cell dysfunction even if there exists IR.

7. Other pathogenic alterations of DM2

7.1 Hyperglucagonemia

It has been found that in DM2 patients, fasting and postprandial glucagon levels are increased and directly correlated to the higher glucose production; such that in DM2 patients, hyperglucagonemia contributes to fasting hyperglycemia through hepatic gluconeogenesis. The bihormonal theory in DM2, insulin deficit and glucagon increase, was proposed in 1981 by Unger and is widely accepted today [35].

7.2 Diminished incretin effect

It has been demonstrated that orally administered glucose induces greater insulin secretion than intravenously injected glucose; this is called the incretin effect.

Incretins are peptides secreted in the digestive tract that have a role in the regulation of glycemia. These are GLP-1 and glucose-dependent insulinotropic polypeptide (GIP). These peptides, synthesized in the ileum and the jejunum, are released after oral glucose intake, stimulating endogenous insulin secretion and reducing glucagon secretion; also, they slow down gastric emptying and reduce appetite. GLP-1 is much more important, contributing with 90% to the total effect.

Decreased incretin effect is associated with the lower GLP-1 levels exhibited by DM2 patients in the postabsorptive state; GLP-1 deficit is related to lower insulin secretion, and consequently glucose production in the liver after meals is not inhibited either [36].

7.3 Microbiota

The digestive tract hosts a complex bacterial ecosystem of nearly 100 trillion microorganisms, with about 1000 species having multiple nutritional and metabolic functions. In DM2 patients, compared with nondiabetic subjects, a proportional increase of Gram-negative bacteria has been found, which would participate in the chronic inflammation state of this pathology [37].

Several mechanisms are proposed to explain the influence of gut microbiota (GM) on the onset of IR and DM2; the best founded mechanism postulated is the change in intestinal permeability with increase of endotoxemia.

It has been observed that since the beginning of the development of obesity and DM2, there exists an alteration in GM that is capable of inducing a disturbance in the intestinal barrier, causing the person to absorb more toxic substances. This metabolic endotoxemia, characterized by an increase in serum levels of lipopolysaccharides, contributes to the low-grade chronic inflammatory state that is associated to IR and to DM2 [38].

Lipopolysaccharides derived from the cell membrane of the Gram-negative bacteria of GM are known inflammation stimulators, which could be explained because they bind to Toll-like receptor 4 (TLR4) present in adipocytes, stimulating the production of proinflammatory cytokines, particularly TNFα and IL-6. These TLR4 favor NF-kβ activation, which regulates the synthesis of inflammatory molecules [39]; activation of TLR4 would cause an increase in the activity of the NF-kβ transcription factors of proinflammatory cytokines which prevent the interaction of insulin with its receptor, contributing to DM2 through lower insulin action.

7.4 Increased renal glucose reabsorption

It is presently accepted that alterations in the renal mechanisms of glucose regulation would be involved in the pathogenesis of DM2. In experimental studies, it has been demonstrated that in DM2 there exists a poor adaptive response of the kidney, through higher renal glucose reabsorption, favoring hyperglycemia [40].

Glucose reabsorption is mediated by sodium glucose-linked transporters (SGLT), a family of membrane transporters widely distributed throughout the body, of which SGLT1 and SGLT2 are expressed in the proximal convoluted tubule of the kidney. SGLT2 has a high capacity and reabsorbs 90% of the filtered glucose; this physiological mechanism is produced through a process of sodium/glucose active cotransport, such that when sodium is absorbed, an energy gradient is produced that permits the entry of glucose into blood circulation independently of insulin [41].

In DM2 patients, a higher synthesis and absorption capacity of SLGT2 have been demonstrated, increasing maximal glucose transport from a glycemia of 180 mg/dl in healthy subjects to 240 mg/dl in DM2 patients. Thus, glucosuria begins at higher glycemic levels, originating a greater glucose reabsorption which contributes to maintaining the hyperglycemia. On the other side in DM2, increased renal gluconeogenesis has been found, resulting in higher glucose production and favoring even more the hyperglycemia of these patients [42].

Considering all the above, in relation to the pathogenesis of DM2, DeFronzo [30] describes what he called the ominous octet, because the alterations exhibited by these patients are eight. These are in pancreatic β cells, less insulin secretion; IR in the liver with increase in gluconeogenesis; IR in muscular tissue with less glucose uptake; IR in adipose tissue with greater FFA production; in the gut, reduction in GLP-1 release with decreased incretin effect; hyperglucagonemia due to greater production in pancreatic α cells; in the kidney, increase in glucose reabsorption; and in the brain, IR with a non-clarified effect.

In 2016, Schwartz [43] published that the alterations in DM2 patients are 11, thus adding to those mentioned above, gut microbiota, deregulation of the immune system, and increase of glucose uptake in the gut. The object of this description is to find similarities between the pathogenesis of DM2 and the pathogenesis of type 1 diabetes and in the future create a new β cell-centric classification of diabetes.

8. Therapeutic implications of the pathogenesis of DM2

The present knowledge on the pathogenesis of DM2 has permitted the development of various drugs for the treatment of this type of diabetes, which act on the different disturbances presented by these patients to correct the multiple pathogenic disorders.

Sulfonylureas (SU), the first drugs used (1954), act on the β cells stimulating insulin secretion by closure of the ATP-sensitive K channels and elevation of intracellular calcium.

Later, in 1997, meglitinides appear they are insulin-secreting drugs with a shorter action than SU, which are employed as prandial regulators of glycemia. Their mechanism of action is similar to that of SU; they bind to specific receptors in the β cells, different from those of SU. Their use has been very limited due to their lower effectiveness and higher cost.

Metformin, introduced in the USA in 1955, is an insulin-sensitizing drug belonging to the biguanide family, widely used as a monodrug or associated with other hypoglycemic drugs. Metformin reduces IR and fasting hyperglycemia by slowing down gluconeogenesis; it also increases glucose uptake by the muscle and favors glucose utilization by the gut. Several mechanisms of action have been postulated; however, they are still not exactly known.

Another group of insulin-sensitizing drugs is constituted by thiazolidinediones (TZD), incorporated into the drug therapy in the year 2000 with the object

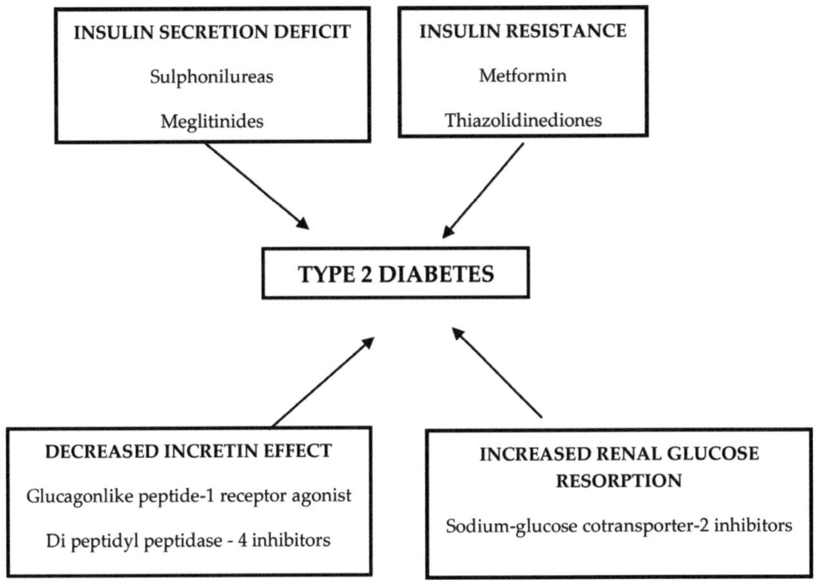

Figure 3.
Pathogenic alterations of type 2 diabetes and pharmacotherapy.

of reducing IR, especially in adipose tissue. They act by binding to the PPAR-ϒ nuclear receptors, also known as glitazone receptors. Their use is restricted and has been questioned because of their adverse effects, among others, heart failure and possible vesical cancer.

In 2005, GLP-1 receptor agonists (GLP-1 RA) were incorporated. These are drugs that improve the diminished incretin effect of DM2 patients. They are resistant to the action of dipeptidyl peptidase-4 (DPP-4) enzyme which degrades native GLP-1 in 1–2 minutes. Through an action similar to GLP-1, they stimulate insulin secretion. GLP-1 RA are injectable and very expensive, and, in addition to their hypoglycemic action, they have other effects as mentioned above.

One year later DPP-4 inhibitors (DPP-4i) appeared, which are at present extensively used. DPP-4i also act restoring the diminished incretin effect; they inhibit the rapid degradation of GLP-1 by the enzyme and indirectly favor insulin secretion.

The most recently incorporated group of hypoglycemic drugs (2013) are the SGLT2 inhibitors that partially block renal glucose reabsorption which is increased in DM2 patients. Their effect is to lower glycemia by causing glucosuria independently of insulin. Several of these drugs are available, and other benefits have been described for them, the most important being a lower risk of cardiovascular disease [45].

Figure 3 shows, together with the main pathogenic alterations of DM2, the corresponding hypoglycemic drugs employed in the usual clinical practice [44].

We hope that in the near future, even better new drugs will be developed that will be able to stop the natural evolution of DM2, slowing down the destruction of the β cell mass and thus reducing the important public health problem of this pathology.

Conflict of interest

The authors declare that they have no conflict of interest associated with this chapter.

Author details

Pilar Durruty[1,2]*, María Sanzana[2] and Lilian Sanhueza[3,4]

1 Diabetes Unit, Department of Medicine, Faculty of Medicine, San Juan de Dios Hospital, University of Chile, Santiago, Chile

2 Endocrinology and Diabetes Section, Department of Medicine, Clinical Hospital of the Faculty of Medicine, University of Chile, Santiago, Chile

3 Diabetes Unit, Internal Medicine Service, San Juan de Dios Hospital, Santiago, Chile

4 Department of Medicine, Faculty of Medical Sciences, University of Santiago of Chile, Santiago, Chile

*Address all correspondence to: padurrutya@yahoo.es

References

[1] Stumvoll M, Goldstein BJ, van Haeften TW. Type 2 diabetes: Principles of pathogenesis and therapy. Lancet. 2005;**365**:1333-1346

[2] Taylor R. Type 2 diabetes: Etiology and reversibility. Diabetes Care. 2013;**36**:1047-1055

[3] Durruty P, Pérez-Bravo F. Patogénesis de la diabetes mellitus. In: García de los Ríos M, Durruty P, editors. Diabetes Mellitus. 3era ed. Santiago, Chile: Editorial Mediterráneo Ltda; 2014. pp. 25-39

[4] Ferranini E, Gastaldelli A, Iozzo P. Pathophysiology of prediabetes. The Medical Clinics of North America. 2011;**95**:327-339

[5] Meigs JB, Cupples LA, Wilson PW. Parental transmission of type 2 diabetes: The Framingham study. Diabetes. 2000;**49**:2201-2207

[6] Ridderstrale M, Groop L. Genetic dissection of type 2 diabetes. Molecular and Cellular Endocrinology. 2009;**297**:10-17

[7] Groop L, Lyssenko V. Genes and type 2 diabetes mellitus. Current Diabetes Reports. 2008;**8**:192-197

[8] Cusi K, Maezono K, Mandarino L. Insulin resistance differentially affect the PI 3-kinase- and MAP kinase-mediated signaling in human muscle. The Journal of Clinical Investigation. 2000;**105**:311-320

[9] Buraczynska M, Wacinski P, Stec A, Kuczmaszewska A. Calpain-10 gene polymorphisms in type 2 diabetes and its micro and macrovascular complications. Journal of Diabetes and its Complications. 2013;**27**:54-58

[10] Kimber CH, Doney AS, Pearson ER, McCarthy MI, Hattersley AT, Leese GP, et al. TCF7L2 in the Go-DARTS study: Evidence for a gene dose effect on both diabetes susceptibility and control of glucose levels. Diabetologia. 2007;**50**:1186-1191

[11] Eckel R, Kahn S, Ferranini E. Obesity and type 2 diabetes: What can be unified and what needs to be individualized? The Journal of Clinical Endocrinology and Metabolism. 2011;**96**:1654-1663

[12] Mujica V. Diabetes en el adulto mayor. In: García de los Ríos M, Durruty P, editors. Diabetes Mellitus. 3era ed. Santiago, Chile: Editorial Mediterráneo Ltda; 2014. pp. 314-325

[13] Tabák AG, Abaraly TN, Batty GD, Kivimäki M. Depression and type 2 diabetes: A causal association? The Lancet Diabetes and Endocrinology. 2014;**2**:236-245

[14] Carnethon MR, Biggs ML, Barzilay JI, Smith NL, Vaccarino V, Bertoni AG, et al. Longitudinal association between depressive symptoms and incident type 2 diabetes mellitus in older adults: The cardiovascular health study. Archives of Internal Medicine. 2007;**167**:802-807

[15] Reutrakul S, Van Cauter E. Interactions between sleep, circadian function, and glucose metabolism: Implications for the risk and severity of diabetes. Annals of the New York Academy of Sciences. 2014;**1311**:151-173

[16] Durruty P, García de los Ríos M. Glucotoxicity and lipotoxicity: Factors in the pathogenesis and evolution of type 2 diabetes. Revista Médica de Chile. 2001;**129**:671-679

[17] Rains JL, Jain SK. Oxidative stress, insulin signalling, and diabetes. Free Radical Biology & Medicine. 2011;**50**:567-575

[18] Mancuso P. The role of adipokines in chronic inflammation. ImmunoTargets and Therapy. 2016;**5**:47-56

[19] Neel BA, Sargis RM. The paradox of progress: Environmental disruption of metabolism and the diabetes epidemic. Diabetes. 2011;**60**:1838-1848

[20] Ghemrawi R, Battaglia-Hsu SF, Arnold C. Endoplasmic reticulum stress in metabolic disorders. Cell. 2018;7:1-35

[21] Bradford BL, Shulman GI. Mitochondrial dysfunction and type 2 diabetes. Science. 2005;**307**:384-387

[22] Mirtschink P, Jang C, Arany Z, Krek W. Fructose metabolism, cardiometabolic risk, and the epidemic of coronary artery disease. European Heart Journal. 2018;**39**:2497-2525

[23] Mirmiran P, Esfandyari S, Moghadam SK, Bahadoran Z, Azizi F. Fatty acid quality and quantity of diet and risk of type 2 diabetes in adults: Tehran lipid and glucose study. Journal of Diabetic Complications. 2018;**32**:655-659

[24] Yerlikaya A, Dagel T, King CH, Kubawara M, Lanaspa MA, Andrés Hernando A, et al. Dietary and commercialized fructose: Sweet or Sour? International Urology and Nephrology. 2017;**49**:1611-1620

[25] Zong G, Lebwohl B, Hu F, Sampson L, Dougherty L, Willet WC, et al. Gluten intake and risk of type 2 diabetes in three large prospective cohort studies of US men and women. Diabetologia. 2018;**61**:2164-2173

[26] Mathieu CH. Vitamin D and diabetes: Where do we stand? Diabetes Research and Clinical Practice. 2015;**108**:201-209

[27] Stumvoll M, Häring H, Fritsche A. For debate: Starling's curve of the pancreas overuse of a concept? Hormone and Metabolic Research. 2003;**35**:391-395

[28] Robertson RP, Harmon J, Tran PO, Tanaka Y, Takahashi H. Glucose toxicity in β-cells: Type 2 diabetes, good radicals gone bad, and the glutathione connection. Diabetes. 2003;**52**:581-587

[29] O'Rahilly S, Turner RC, Mathews DR. Impaired pulsatile secretion of insulin in relatives of patients with non insulin-dependent diabetes. The New England Journal of Medicine. 1988;**318**:1225-1230

[30] DeFronzo RA. From the triumvirate to the ominous octet: A new paradigm for the treatment of type 2 diabetes mellitus. Diabetes. 2009;**58**:773-795

[31] Hayden M. Islet amyloid, metabolic syndrome, and the natural progressive history of type 2 diabetes mellitus. Journal of the Pancreas. 2002;**3**:126-138

[32] Yokoi N. Epigenetic dysregulation in pancreatic islets and pathogenesis of type 2 diabetes. Journal of Diabetes Investigation. 2018;**9**:475-477

[33] Bogardus C, Lillioja S, Stone K. Correlation between glycogen synthase activity and in vivo insulin action in man. The Journal of Clinical Investigation. 1984;**73**:1185-1900

[34] Draznin B. Molecular mechanisms of insulin resistance: Serine phosphorylation of insulin receptor substrate-1 and increased expression of p85alpha: The two sides of a coin. Diabetes. 2006;**55**:2392-2397

[35] Unger RH, Orci L. Glucagon and the cell physiology and pathophysiology. The New England Journal of Medicine. 1981;**304**:1518-1524

[36] Drucker DJ, Nauck MA. The incretin system: Glucagon-like peptide-1 receptor agonists and dipeptidyl

peptidase-4 inhibitors in type 2 diabetes. Lancet. 2006;**368**:1696-1705

[37] Muñoz-Garach A, Díaz-Perdigones C, Tinahones FJ. Gut microbiota and type 2 diabetes mellitus. Endocrinología y Nutrición. 2016;**63**:560-568

[38] Cani P, Bibiloni R, Knauf C, Waget A, Neyrinck A, Delzenne N. Changes in gut microbiota control metabolic endotoxemia-induced inflammation in high-fat diet-induced obesity and diabetes in mice. Diabetes. 2008;**57**:1470-1481

[39] Pussinen P, Havulinna A, Lehto M, Sundvall J, Salomaa V. Endotoxemia is associated with an increased risk of incident diabetes. Diabetes Care. 2011;**34**:392-397

[40] Abdul-Ghani M, Norton L, DeFronzo R. Role of sodium-glucose cotransporter 2 (SGLT 2) inhibitors in the treatment of type 2 diabetes. Endocrine Reviews. 2011;**32**:515-531

[41] Wright E, Hirayama B, Loo F. Active sugar transport in health and disease. Journal of Internal Medicine. 2007;**261**:32-43

[42] Bakris G, Fonseca V, Sharma K, Wright E. Renal sodium–glucose transport: Role in diabetes mellitus and potential clinical implications. Kidney International. 2009;**75**:1272-1277

[43] Schwartz S, Epstein S, Corkey B, Grant S, Gavin J, Aguilar R. The time is right for a classification system for diabetes: Rationale and implications of the b-cell–centric classification schema. Diabetes Care. 2016;**39**:179-186

[44] Standars of Medical Care in Diabetes 2018 (ADA). Pharmacologic approaches to glycemic treatment. Diabetes Care. 2018;**41**(Suppl. 1): S73-S85

[45] Zelniker TA, Wivioytt SD, Raz I, Im K, Goodrich EL, Bonaca MP, et al. SGLT2 inhibitors for primary and secondary prevention of cardiovascular and renal outcomes in type 2 diabetes: A systematic review and meta-analysis of cardiovascular outcomes trials. The Lancet. 2018;**393**:31-39. DOI: 10.1016/S0140-6736(18)32590-X

Chapter 3

Oxidative Stress, DNA Damage and Repair Pathways in Patients with Type 2 Diabetes Mellitus

Jessica E.B.F. Lima, Danilo J. Xavier and Elza T. Sakamoto-Hojo

Abstract

Type 2 diabetes mellitus (T2D) is characterized mainly by insulin resistance and/or deficiency, presenting risk factors related to aging, hypercaloric diet and sedentary lifestyle. Hyperglycemia, a hallmark of T2D, contributes significantly to the production of reactive oxygen species (ROS), inducing oxidative stress and various cellular and molecular changes in the body. As a consequence, several signaling pathways may be affected, mainly involving biological processes such as inflammation, DNA damage responses, antioxidant defense and metabolic changes. All these processes are relevant for the understanding of the pathogenesis of T2D, and also for the development of diabetic complications in chronic patients. Recently, common characteristics linking T2D to Alzheimer's disease (AD) have been reported. The purpose of this chapter is to highlight the main processes associated with the disease, such as insulin signaling pathways, oxidative stress, mitochondrial dysfunction, DNA damage and repair and antioxidant defense. In addition, the molecular impact of nutritional interventions in patients with T2D will also be addressed, as will the molecular keystones linking T2D and AD. Recently, there is accumulated evidence indicating that the two diseases may share common signaling pathways that may be relevant to the etiopathogenesis of each of them.

Keywords: type 2 diabetes mellitus, insulin resistance, hyperglycemia, oxidative stress, DNA repair, reactive oxygen species (ROS), mitochondrial dysfunction, Alzheimer's disease

1. Introduction

Diabetes mellitus is a metabolic disease that has a major impact on global public health, affecting more than 425 million people worldwide. The number of affected people tends to increase, mainly due to obesity, a risk factor closely related to type 2 diabetes mellitus (T2D), the most common form of diabetes. Hyperglycemia is the most striking feature of the disease, which is the increase of blood glucose levels above those presented by healthy individuals. This could be the main consequence of poor insulin secretion, lack of insulin sensitivity in target tissues or the combination of both [1, 2].

The genetic predisposition may be one of the determinants that favor the susceptibility to T2D development. Several variants of genes and even epigenetic modifications in histones and DNA methylation may influence the heritability of T2D [3, 4]. Due to the complexity of the interaction of different factors involved in this disease, genome-wide association studies (GWAS) have been performed in an attempt to identify genetic variants related to the increased risk of T2D.

In 2007, the first GWAS was performed in France in patients with T2D [5]; At present, at least 75 associated loci have been identified, including the *TCF7L2* transcription factor, which is the most common gene found, in addition to *PPARG, KCNJ11, FTO, CDKN2A/2B, CDKAL1, IGFBP2* among others [6]. Since then, similar studies showed that the loci presenting greater association with T2D vary as regards the relative risk between different ethnicities [7]. Besides, these variants explain only a low percentage of the disease heritability, most of which are found in intergenic or intronic regions [6]. Furthermore, DNA methylation patterns may contribute to genetic susceptibility to T2D. There is evidence of an increased risk of T2D development associated with distinct methylation patterns in some loci [8], but this approach is still a major challenge for researchers.

While obesity and overweight have been considered an important cause of T2D, a poor diet and lack of physical activity significantly contribute to an increased risk of insulin resistance and T2D [9].

One of the greatest concerns regarding the poor glycemic control in patients with T2D is related to the micro and macrovascular complications of diabetes. Since the onset of T2D did not present specific acute symptoms, 50% of adults with T2D do not know that they have the disease [9]. Chronic hyperglycemia induces a series of complications, such as retinopathy, neuropathy and nephropathy. In a long term, the high blood glucose levels may also induce endothelial dysfunction, which contributes to the increased risk for the development of cardiovascular diseases.

2. Oxidative stress and mitochondrial dysfunction

Changes in glucose homeostasis represent a critical factor for the development of metabolic diseases. Normally, to maintain optimal levels of blood glucose, the pancreas secretes two hormones. In response to high glucose levels, pancreatic β cells secrete insulin, which promote the uptake of glucose by peripheral tissues, reduce gluconeogenesis and decrease glycogen and triglyceride breakdown. However, when glucose levels are reduced in the blood, α-cells release glucagon, which will reverse the above process.

Overall, insulin resistance is one of the main causes of disturbances in glucose homeostasis; when insulin receptors do not respond to the amount of insulin produced, the consequence is a deficiency of the body in the glucose uptake and absorption. As a compensatory mechanism, pancreatic β cells increase the release of insulin, but if the glucose levels remain high due to the inability of insulin to achieve body's demand, it may occur the onset of T2D. Insulin resistance persists in patients since pre-diabetes, a stage in which individuals show glucose levels above the normal values, but not so high for the diagnosis of the disease. It should be mention that at this stage, a healthy nutritional style, physical exercises and weight control may allow the individuals to recover normal glucose levels.

At a long term, high levels of blood glucose can lead to a number of cellular and molecular changes in the body, especially due to the production of reactive oxygen species (ROS) [10]. It is well known that mitochondria are the main source of ROS; these highly dynamic organelles constantly undergo structural changes, responding rapidly to the physiological alterations in the environment. Exposure of cells to hyperglycemic conditions is associated with several mitochondrial alterations. There is evidence that the number and morphology of mitochondria are essential for the maintenance of cellular function. Hyperglycemia in this context is reported as an inducer of glucose metabolism, which can promote several conformational changes in mitochondria, overload of the electron transport chain, leading to the overproduction of ROS, and mitochondrial dysfunction [11–14].

It has been reported [15] that patients with pre-diabetes presented an increase in the mitochondrial mass, suggesting that the initial increase in blood glucose levels may induce an adaptative response in order to increase mitochondrial biogenesis to maintain homeostasis. These results are associated with an increase in mitophagy, raising evidence that during pre-diabetes state there may be an elimination of compromised mitochondria in an attempt to reduce mitochondrial oxidative stress [15, 16].

ROS are normal byproducts of aerobic respiration, consisting of non-radicals, as hydrogen peroxide (H_2O_2) and free radicals, as hydroxyl radical (OH) and superoxide anion (O_2^-). In normal situations, antioxidant enzymes (glutathione peroxidase, catalase and superoxide dismutase) are able to eliminate ROS and maintain the homeostasis of the organism. However, in a hyperglycemic state, the mitochondria electron transport chain becomes hyperactive, thus inducing an excessive production of ROS that surpasses the antioxidant defense system [17]. The imbalance between the prooxidants and the antioxidant defense system lead to a condition called oxidative stress, where the reactive molecules can cause damage to lipids, proteins and nucleic acids [18].

Among DNA damage caused by ROS, the major oxidized base modifications generated are 8-oxoguanine (8-oxoG) and 8-oxodesoxyguanosine (8-oxodG), which could occur in both DNA and the nucleotide pool, the latter can be incorporated into the DNA during replication or repair [19, 20]. The repair of 8-oxoG in DNA is performed by the base excision repair mechanism (BER), in which the DNA glycosylase OGG1 recognizes the 8oxoG and together with APE1 enzyme, polymerase complex β and DNA ligase I promote DNA repair [21, 22]; the removal of 8-oxo-dG from the nucleotide pool is performed by the enzyme hMTH1 (human MutT homolog), which hydrolyses 8-oxo-dGTP to transport this molecule to the cytosol, preventing its incorporation into the DNA [23]. For different types of DNA lesions, other DNA repair processes, such as nucleotide excision, homologous recombination, non-homologous end-joining, and mismatch repair may also occur. In diabetes, there is evidence that DNA repair levels and activity of antioxidant enzymes are reduced [24, 25], as well as DNA damage levels and oxidized bases in these patients were found increased [26, 27].

The oxidative stress promoted by chronic hyperglycemia causes cellular damage mainly in the pancreatic β cells, which present low levels of antioxidant enzymes, and are more susceptible to damages caused by ROS. This stress is also responsible for releasing inflammatory mediators, which in turn culminate in a vicious cycle leading to β-cell dysfunction, insulin resistance and metabolic decline, which are critical for the development of T2D [28].

In diabetes, high glucose levels may also induce endoplasmic reticulum (ER) stress. Since the ER is the main responsible for protein maturation and folding, in particular proinsulin, in a hyperglycemic state, this molecule tends to be excessively synthesized and can overload the ER, leading to the accumulation of misfolded proteins, thus generating a stress condition. This stress may lead to the activation of the unfolded protein response pathway, which may restore ER homeostasis or induce cell death. The latter may lead to β-cell dysfunction, and consequently, to the reduction of insulin secretion and chronic hyperglycemia [28–31].

Several metabolic pathways are involved in insulin resistance and induction of inflammation and stress, including the JNK (JUN N-terminal kinase) and IKKβ (IκB kinase-β) pathways, both of them can be activated by ER stress [32]. IKKβ is a protein responsible for mediating the activation of NF-κβ (nuclear factor-κB), which in turn stimulates the proinflammatory cytokines, TNF-α (tumor necrosis factor-alpha) and interleukin 1β (IL-1β), that can promote inhibition of the insulin receptor substrate (IRS) protein phosphorylation or reduce their transcriptional expression, compromising the insulin pathway and contributing to insulin resistance [25, 28].

Obesity is another critical factor that results in oxidative stress and insulin resistance [33], generating a chronic inflammatory condition in adipose tissue, causing the recurrent release of pro-inflammatory cytokines, such as those previously mentioned, in addition to interleukin 6 (IL-6), which together lead to pancreatic β-cell dysfunction, decreased insulin secretion, and consequently hyperglycemia and thus triggering T2D [28].

3. Insulin signaling pathway

The normal signalization of the insulin signaling pathway is vital and its dysregulation is implicated not only in T2D but also in diseases such as cancer, cardiovascular and neurodegenerative diseases. Changes in this signaling cascade as well as the consequences thereof, makes this pathway an important subject of study, considering its relevance in terms of age-related diseases.

Normally, the transport of glucose into the cells occurs through different intracellular signaling mechanisms performed in cascade, as shown in **Figure 1**. Firstly, insulin binds to its receptor, promoting tyrosine phosphorylation of IRS proteins, especially IRS-1 and 2. The tyrosine phosphorylation is critical for the

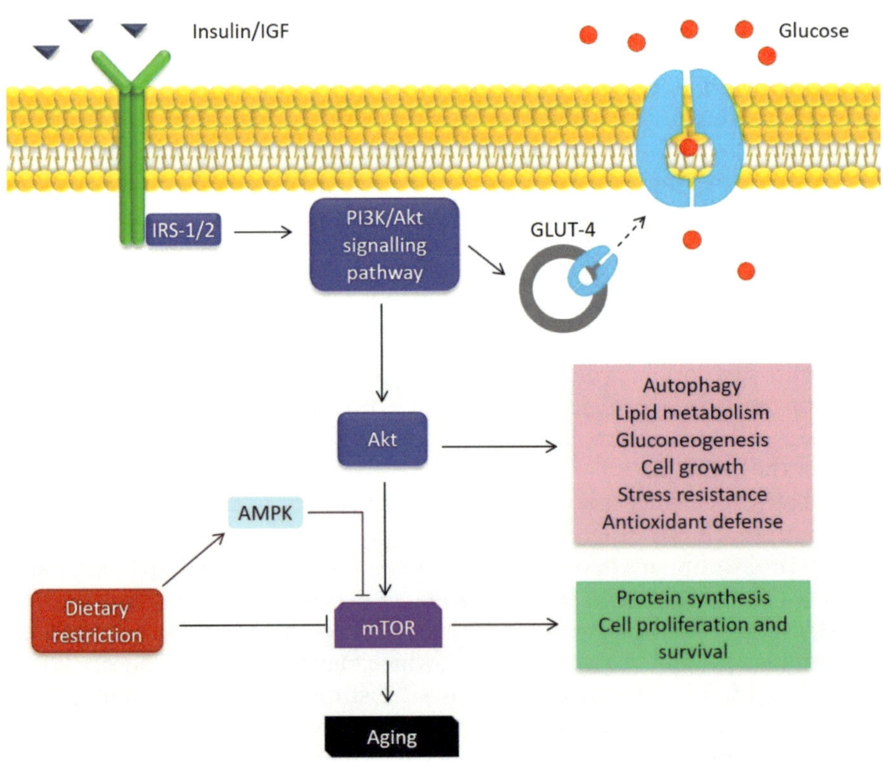

Figure 1.
Insulin/insulin-like growth factor signaling pathway.

correct activation of the insulin pathway. Phosphorylation at serine or threonine residues is associated with the inhibition or even degradation of IRS proteins promoting downregulation of the pathway. This inhibitory effect over the pathway occurs normally via insulin-induced kinases as a way to keep the correct function of all proteins involved. However, some conditions as hyperglycemia, release of proinflammatory cytokines, oxidative stress (due to mitochondrial dysfunction), in addition to elevated fatty acids and ER stress can induce an increased serine or threonine phosphorylation, promoting the downregulation of insulin signaling and exacerbating the insulin resistance condition [2, 34, 35].

Thus, tyrosine phosphorylation of IRS proteins, further activate PI3K (phosphatidylinositol 3-kinase) protein [36, 37], promoting in particular the translocation of glucose transporter 4 (GLUT4) to the plasma membrane enabling the entrance of glucose into the cell [38]. Among the PI3K-associated downstream proteins, here we focus especially on Akt (alpha serine/threonine-protein kinase) [39, 40]. Once activated, Akt-regulated proteins have a key role in metabolism, glycogen synthesis, autophagy, growth, cell survival, transcription and protein synthesis [41]. Akt has been described as an important downregulator of GSK3α/β proteins. These proteins are strongly associated with the formation of amyloid beta and phosphorylation of tau protein, which are the main proteins involved in Alzheimer's disease [42, 43]. Another important target of Akt are the FOXO (Forkhead box O) transcription factors, which regulates the expression of different genes related to gluconeogenesis, lipid metabolism, resistance to stress, DNA repair, cell growth, survival, differentiation, among others [41, 44, 45]. The kinase mTOR (mammalian target of rapamycin), responsible for regulating cell growth and metabolism, being a large sensor of nutrients and cellular energy, is also a target of Akt [46–48] and has a major role in the mechanism of longevity extension [49].

There is evidence that changes in the expression of growth factors, IRS proteins, IGF-1, AKT, mTOR, FOXO among others that result in downregulation of the insulin signaling pathway through nutritional restriction, for example, are implicated in the resistance to stress, induction of autophagy, extension of longevity and reduction of aging-related diseases in different species, such as worms, flies, rats, mice and some primates [47, 50–55]. The inhibition of mTOR has been widely discussed as the main protein involved in the longevity extension. Metformin, a drug commonly used to control the glycemic levels in diabetics, is able to inhibit the activity of mTOR, via activation of AMPK, a protein with role in glycolysis, fatty acid oxidation, lipogenesis reduction, gluconeogenesis and protein synthesis [52, 56, 57]. AMPK is also important in mitochondrial biogenesis, since it activates PGC1α [58], which has the ability to stimulate the mitochondrial electron transport chain and suppress ROS levels, being essential in inducing the antioxidant defense system [49, 59].

4. Impact of nutritional interventions in diabetes care

Diabetes is a global health problem. Currently, the treatment of this disease has been carried out with medications, such as metformin, aiming to reduce the blood glucose levels, in an attempt to prevent a series of alterations in the cellular metabolism caused by chronic hyperglycemia. However, the success of treatments, in general, is limited, requiring other types of interventions (nutritional and regular physical activity, mainly) related to the patients' lifestyle. The majority of patients with T2D present age between 40 and 59 years, which is critical for the disease [9] and in this phase, as in the subsequent stages, with the progression of the aging process, the protein homeostasis becomes increasingly compromised, also accompanied by a reduction in the efficiency of the DNA repair system and the antioxidant defense, besides the organism as a whole, consequently leading to the accumulation of cellular damage [51, 58, 60, 61].

A great number of patients with T2D are overweight or obese. Changes in the lifestyle have been shown essential in controlling the levels of blood glucose. Additionally, it was reported that T2D patients submitted to a 7-day intervention to achieve adequate blood glucose levels led to a significant decrease in DNA damage levels [26]. In particular, some nutritional interventions, as well as caloric (CR) or protein restriction, have been shown to be very effective, not only for reducing blood glucose levels, but also for having very positive benefits in terms of increased life expectancy, as demonstrated in several model organisms [52, 54], in addition to reducing the incidence of aging-related diseases [62–64].

A major recruitment study known as CALERIE (Comprehensive Assessment of Long-term Effects of Reducing Intake of Energy) aimed to show the effects of caloric restriction in humans. It has already been shown that in a period of 2 years, the CR is very efficient in improving insulin sensitivity [65], reducing inflammatory markers [66] and reducing oxidative stress [67]. Those features are especially significantly increased in patients with T2D, which would make this approach a valuable intervention for treatment of those patients. In fact, in a study performed in rhesus monkeys, from the 38 control animals, 16 developed high levels of blood glucose, becoming either prediabetic or diabetic. On the other hand, all the animals under caloric restriction did not present any impairment on glucose regulation [64], which may demonstrate the importance of this kind of intervention.

Although this approach has been widely discussed, the studies are still controversial regarding the best diet composition for diabetic patients. It has been hypothesized that a high intake of proteins could influence the effects of a caloric restriction [68]. In fact, there is a study showing the efficiency of a protein restriction intervention on reducing cancer incidence and extending lifespan regardless the intake of calories [69].

5. Susceptibility of T2D to Alzheimer's disease

Alzheimer's disease (AD) is a progressive, continuous neurodegenerative disorder that affects large areas of the cerebral cortex and hippocampus. These abnormalities are usually detected for the first time in brain tissue involving the frontal and temporal lobes and then slowly advance to other areas of the neocortex at rates that vary considerably between individuals [70]. By 2018, an estimated 50 million people are living with dementia, with AD being the most prevalent form [71]. The main symptoms of AD result from the formation of beta-amyloid (Aβ) plaques and neurofibrillary tangles of the tau protein in the brain, which together lead to neuronal dysfunction and death, causing memory loss episodes which are characteristic of the pathology [70, 72]. It has been reported that similar to the toxicity caused by Aβ aggregates in the brains of patients with AD, amyloid deposits in the pancreas occur in patients with diabetes, which may induce the death of pancreatic insulin-producing β cells [73].

Recently, several studies have narrowed the relationship between T2D and dementias [74, 75], suggesting that in addition to an increase in the incidence of dementia in T2D patients, a more rapid cognitive decline may also occur, including a higher conversion rate of individuals who have mild cognitive impairment in patients with dementia [76–78]. This information has aroused interest in studying a possible association between T2D and dementia.

Many hypotheses have been raised about the common features that involve the two pathologies and how these can be related to each other. It has been suggested that both diseases may share common signaling pathways, although molecular and cellular mechanisms still need elucidation. There is evidence that insulin resistance in the brain, including insulin pathway dysregulation, inflammatory processes, formation of advanced glycation products, as well as oxidative stress and mitochondrial dysfunction, may be implicated in the pathogenesis of AD and T2D [79].

Insulin, besides having an essential role as regulator of energy metabolism, also exerts a role in plasticity, survival and neuronal growth, as well as learning and memory processes, contributing to the improvement of cognitive functions; their absence has been associated with cognitive decline in patients with neurological and neurodegenerative diseases, such as AD [80–82]. In fact, it has been demonstrated that brains of patients with AD present altered insulin signaling [83]. Insulin receptors are found in the central nervous system (CNS) in large number and their impairment (hence the signaling cascade) may culminate in a number of alterations mainly involving PI3K, AKT and mTOR proteins. Abnormal expression of these and other proteins and the deregulation of this pathway may contribute to the formation of Aβ aggregates, neurofibrillary tangles by hyperphosphorylation of the tau protein [84], as well as the impairment of the autophagy process regulated by mTOR [75], whose hyperexpression has been related to T2D [85] and AD [86].

Thus, in the same way as T2D, AD is a disease related to less efficient molecular signaling in response to insulin, inflammation, oxidative stress, formation of advanced glycation end products and increased accumulation of DNA damage [87–89]. Thus, these characteristics suggest a connection between the two diseases.

The presence of higher levels of inflammation has already been described both in T2D and AD patients. In T2D there is a chronic inflammatory response localized in adipose tissue and characterized by the infiltration of immune system components, mainly macrophages, which release different proinflammatory cytokines such as TNF-α and IL-6 [90, 91]. Such cytokines may lead to insulin resistance by inducing cytokine signaling suppressors (SOCS), which participate in the degradation of IRS-1 and IRS-2 [92, 93]. In addition, these cytokines also activate stress response kinases, such as JNK and NF-κβ, which in turn act on the insulin receptor, inhibiting its tyrosine kinase activity, therefore culminating in insulin resistance [94, 95].

Similar inflammatory processes probably occur in the brain and peripheral tissues. Several studies have established the presence of inflammatory markers in the brains of patients with AD, including high levels of cytokines/chemokines [96]. In addition, inflammatory mediator levels in blood as TNF-α, IL-6 and IL-1b are increased in AD patients [97]. Thus, both in the brain and in peripheral tissues, chronic inflammation becomes harmful, leading to progressive damage to tissues and consequently triggering degenerative diseases.

There is evidence that insulin plays an important role in glucose regulation in the CNS, and its additional effects on neurons include metabolic, neurotrophic, neuromodulatory and neuroendocrine actions [98]. The presence of higher levels of inflammatory mediators in the CNS seems to stimulate the formation of beta-amyloid oligomers and neurofibrillary tangles, which trigger the removal of insulin receptors in neurons, making this condition common in both T2D and AD, triggering progression of both diseases [89, 99] (**Figure 2**).

Besides, the lower sensitivity to insulin, in addition to being important for the progression of T2D, also appears to affect the expression and metabolism of Aβ proteins in the CNS, and consequently, an increase in oxidative stress condition [2, 100], which in turn, induces greater accumulation of Aβ oligomers [101] and the release of inflammatory mediators [88], as already mentioned. Thus, it seems

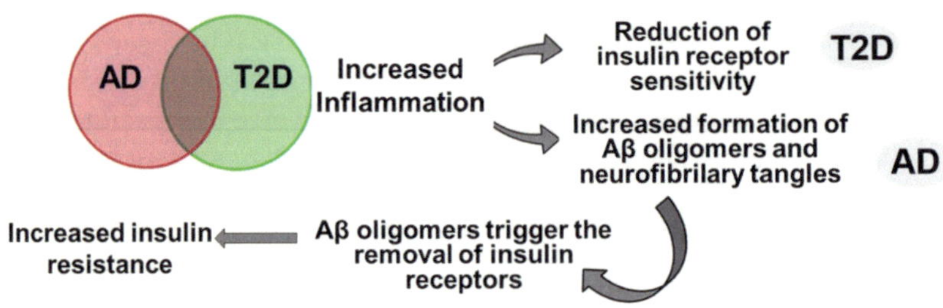

Figure 2.
Relationship between increased levels of inflammatory factors and insulin sensitivity in both diseases, T2D and AD. Increased insulin resistance will lead to disease progression and the development of comorbidities in both T2D and AD.

that all these processes are related to T2D and AD as a vicious cycle, leading to the development and progression of comorbidities in both diseases, being one of the consequences of hyperglycemia and the accumulation of Aβ oligomers, respectively.

However, both diseases seem to present less efficient DNA repair processes, which generate genomic instability and also cell death; this condition is closely related to the complications reported for patients with T2D, and also AD [24, 102]. According to Xavier et al. [103], hyperglycemic T2D patients presented induction of DNA repair pathways, probably in response to higher levels of oxidative stress, but it remains to be elucidated whether the efficacy of repair pathways are normal in non-hyperglycemic T2D patients. In the case of AD, there is evidence that repair of DNA double strand breaks is less efficient [104], as well as base excision repair pathway [105], which would be detrimental to AD individuals, considering the relevance of DNA repair mechanisms for the DNA damage repair caused by ROS [106], and also by several kinds of endogenous and exogenous agents.

6. Conclusions

Insulin resistance is one of the main causes of disturbances in glucose homeostasis. In patients with T2D, long term exposure to high levels of blood glucose can lead to a number of cellular and molecular changes in the body. In this context, hyperglycemia can promote several conformational changes in mitochondria, overload of the electron transport chain, leading to the overproduction of ROS, and mitochondrial dysfunction. Furthermore, the imbalance between the prooxidant and the antioxidant defense system lead to a condition of oxidative stress, where the reactive molecules can cause damage to lipids, proteins and nucleic acids. Interestingly, there is evidence that DNA repair levels and activity of antioxidant enzymes are reduced in T2D; in the opposite, DNA damage levels as well as oxidized bases in these patients were found increased. Insulin resistance has been also associated with several metabolic pathways and induction of inflammation and stress, including ER stress. Therefore, the normal signalization of the insulin pathway is vital and its dysregulation is implicated not only in T2D but also in other diseases such as cancer, cardiovascular and neurodegenerative diseases. In the brain, there is also evidence of insulin resistance and dysregulation of insulin pathway, generating inflammatory processes, as well as oxidative stress and mitochondrial dysfunction, all of them might be implicated in the pathogenesis of T2D and AD, thus linking the two diseases.

Acknowledgements

Research supported by Coordination for the Improvement of Higher Education Personnel (CAPES), National Council for Scientific and Technological Development (CNPq) and São Paulo Research Foundation (FAPESP). We thank CNPq for providing fellowship to J.E.B.F.Lima.

Conflict of interest

There is no conflict of interests.

Author details

Jessica E.B.F. Lima[1], Danilo J. Xavier[1] and Elza T. Sakamoto-Hojo[1,2]*

1 Department of Genetics, Ribeirão Preto Medical School, University of São Paulo (USP), Ribeirão Preto, SP, Brazil

2 Department of Biology, Faculty of Philosophy, Sciences and Letters at Ribeirão Preto, University of São Paulo (USP), Ribeirão Preto, SP, Brazil

*Address all correspondence to: etshojo@usp.br

References

[1] Taylor SI. Deconstructing type 2 diabetes. Cell. 1999;**97**(1):9-12

[2] DeFronzo RA, Ferrannini E, Groop L, Henry RR, Herman WH, Holst JJ, et al. Type 2 diabetes mellitus. Nature Reviews. Disease Primers. 2015;**1**:15019

[3] Ali O. Genetics of type 2 diabetes. World Journal of Diabetes. 2013;**4**(4):114

[4] Basile KJ, Johnson ME, Xia Q, Grant SFA. Genetic susceptibility to type 2 diabetes and obesity: Follow-up of findings from genome-wide association studies. International Journal of Endocrinology. 2014;**2014**:769671

[5] Sladek R, Rocheleau G, Rung J, Dina C, Shen L, Serre D, et al. A genome-wide association study identifies novel risk loci for type 2 diabetes. Nature. 2007;**445**(7130):881-885

[6] Kwak SH, Park KS. Recent progress in genetic and epigenetic research on type 2 diabetes. Experimental & Molecular Medicine. 2016;**48**(3):e220

[7] Basile KJ, Johnson ME, Xia Q, Grant SFA. Genetic susceptibility to type 2 diabetes and obesity: Follow-up of findings from genome-wide association studies. International Journal of Endocrinology. 2014;**2014**:769671

[8] Chambers JC, Loh M, Lehne B, Drong A, Kriebel J, Motta V, et al. Epigenome-wide association of DNA methylation markers in peripheral blood from Indian Asians and Europeans with incident type 2 diabetes: A nested case-control study. The Lancet Diabetes and Endocrinology. 2015;**3**(7):526-534

[9] International Diabetes Federation. IDF Diabetes Atlas. 8th ed. Brussels, Belgium: International Diabetes Federation; 2017. p. 46

[10] Evans JL, Goldfine ID, Maddux BA, Grodsky GM. Oxidative stress and stress-activated signaling pathways: A unifying hypothesis of type 2 diabetes. Endocrine Reviews. 2002;**23**(5):599-622

[11] Yu T, Robotham JL, Yoon Y. Increased production of reactive oxygen species in hyperglycemic conditions requires dynamic change of mitochondrial morphology. Proceedings of the National Academy of Sciences of the United States of America. 2006;**103**(8):2653-2658

[12] Kauffman ME, Kauffman MK, Traore K, Zhu H, Trush MA, Jia Z. et al., MitoSOX-based flow cytometry for detecting mitochondrial ROS. React Oxyg species (Apex, NC). 2016;**2**(5):361-370

[13] Connolly NMC, Theurey P, Adam-Vizi V, Bazan NG, Bernardi P, Bolaños JP, et al. Guidelines on experimental methods to assess mitochondrial dysfunction in cellular models of neurodegenerative diseases. Cell Death and Differentiation. 2017;**25**(3):542-572

[14] Shah GN, Morofuji Y, Banks WA, Price TO. High glucose-induced mitochondrial respiration and reactive oxygen species in mouse cerebral pericytes is reversed by pharmacological inhibition of mitochondrial carbonic anhydrases: Implications for cerebral microvascular disease in diabetes. Biochemical and Biophysical Research Communications. 2013;**440**(2):354-358

[15] Bhansali S, Bhansali A, Walia R, Saikia UN, Dhawan V. Alterations in mitochondrial oxidative stress and mitophagy in subjects with prediabetes and type 2 diabetes mellitus. Front Endocrinol (Lausanne). 2017;**8**:347

[16] Widlansky ME, Wang J, Shenouda SM, Hagen TM, Smith AR,

Kizhakekuttu TJ, et al. Altered mitochondrial membrane potential, mass, and morphology in the mononuclear cells of humans with type 2 diabetes. Translational Research. 2010;**156**(1):15-25

[17] Hurrle S, Hsu WH. The etiology of oxidative stress in insulin resistance. Biomedical Journal. 2017;**40**(5):257-262

[18] Zhang J, Wang X, Vikash V, Ye Q, Wu D, Liu Y, et al. ROS and ROS-mediated cellular signaling. Oxidative Medicine and Cellular Longevity. 2016;**2016**:4350965

[19] Haghdoost S, Czene S, Näslund I, Skog S, Harms-Ringdahl M. Extracellular 8-oxo-dG as a sensitive parameter for oxidative stress in vivo and in vitro. Free Radical Research. 2005;**39**(2):153-162

[20] Haghdoost S, Sjölander L, Czene S, Harms-Ringdahl M. The nucleotide pool is a significant target for oxidative stress. Free Radical Biology & Medicine. 2006;**41**(4):620-626

[21] Fortini P, Pascucci B, Parlanti E, D'Errico M, Simonelli V, Dogliotti E. 8-Oxoguanine DNA damage: At the crossroad of alternative repair pathways. Mutation Research: Fundamental and Molecular Mechanisms of Mutagenesis. 2003;**531**(1-2):127-139

[22] Almeida KH, Sobol RW. A unified view of base excision repair: Lesion-dependent protein complexes regulated by post-translational modification. DNA Repair (Amst). 2007;**6**(6):695-711

[23] Sangsuwan T, Haghdoost S. The nucleotide pool, a target for low-dose γ-ray-induced oxidative stress. Radiation Research. 2008;**170**(6):776-783

[24] Blasiak J, Arabski M, Krupa R, Wozniak K, Zadrozny M, Kasznicki J, et al. DNA damage and repair in type 2 diabetes mellitus. Mutation Research-Fundamental and Molecular Mechanisms of Mutagenesis. 2004;**554**(1-2):297-304

[25] Tilg H, Moschen A. Inflammatory mechanisms in the regulation of insulin resistance. Molecular Medicine. 2008;**14**(3-4):222-231

[26] Xavier DJ, Takahashi P, Manoel-Caetano FS, Foss-Freitas MC, Foss MC, Donadi EA, et al. One-week intervention period led to improvements in glycemic control and reduction in DNA damage levels in patients with type 2 diabetes mellitus. Diabetes Research and Clinical Practice. 2014;**105**(3):356-363

[27] Sun J, Lou X, Wang H, Sollazzo A, Harms-Ringdahl M, Skog S, et al. Serum 8-hydroxy-2′-deoxyguanosine (8-oxo-dG) levels are elevated in diabetes patients. International Journal of Diabetes in Developing Countries. 2015;**35**(3):368-373

[28] Akash MSH, Rehman K, Chen S. Role of inflammatory mechanisms in pathogenesis of type 2 diabetes mellitus. Journal of Cellular Biochemistry. 2013;**114**(3):525-531

[29] Fonseca SG, Gromada J, Urano F. Endoplasmic reticulum stress and pancreatic beta-cell death. Trends in Endocrinology and Metabolism. 2011;**22**(7):266-274

[30] Dufey E, Sepulveda D, Rojas-Rivera D, Hetz C. Cellular mechanisms of endoplasmic reticulum stress signaling in health and disease. 1. An overview. American journal of physiology. Cell physiology. 2014;**307**(7):C582-C594

[31] Manie SN, Lebeau J, Chevet E. Cellular mechanisms of endoplasmic reticulum stress signaling in health and disease. 3. Orchestrating the unfolded protein response in

oncogenesis: An update. American Journal of Physiology. Cell Physiology. 2014;**307**(10):C901-C907

[32] Hotamisligil GS. Endoplasmic reticulum stress and the inflammatory basis of metabolic disease. Cell. 2010;**140**(6):900-917

[33] Maiese K. New insights for oxidative stress and diabetes mellitus. Oxidative Medicine and Cellular Longevity 2015;**2015**(Dm):46-49

[34] Henriksen EJ, Diamond-Stanic MK, Marchionne EM. Oxidative stress and the etiology of insulin resistance and type 2 diabetes. Free Radical Biology & Medicine. 2011;**51**(5):993-999

[35] Boucher J, Kleinridders A, Kahn CR. Insulin receptor signaling in normal. Cold Spring Harbor Perspectives in Biology. 2014;**6**:a009191

[36] Freude S, Schilbach K, Schubert M. The role of IGF-1 receptor and insulin receptor signaling for the pathogenesis of Alzheimer's disease: From model organisms to human disease. Current Alzheimer Research. 2009;**6**:213-223

[37] Murrow BA, Hoehn KL. Mitochondrial regulation of insulin action. The International Journal of Biochemistry & Cell Biology. 2010;**42**(12):1936-1939

[38] Rochette L, Zeller M, Cottin Y, Vergely C. Diabetes, oxidative stress and therapeutic strategies. Biochimica et Biophysica Acta—General Subjects. 2014;**1840**(9):2709-2729

[39] Sasaoka T, Wada T, Tsuneki H. Lipid phosphatases as a possible therapeutic target in cases of type 2 diabetes and obesity. Pharmacology & Therapeutics. 2006;**112**(3):799-809

[40] Erneux C, Edimo WE, Deneubourg L, Pirson I. SHIP2 multiple functions: A balance between a negative control of PtdIns(3,4,5)P_3 level, a positive control of PtdIns(3,4)P_2 production, and intrinsic docking properties. Journal of Cellular Biochemistry. 2011;**112**(9):2203-2209

[41] Cheng Z, Tseng Y, White MF. Insulin signaling meets mitochondria in metabolism. Trends in Endocrinology and Metabolism. 2010;**21**(10):589-598

[42] Phiel CJ. Wilson C a, Lee VM-Y, Klein PS. GSK-3alpha regulates production of Alzheimer's disease amyloid-beta peptides. Nature. 2003;**423**(lane 2):435-439

[43] Rankin CA, Sun Q, Gamblin TC. Tau phosphorylation by GSK-3β promotes tangle-like filament morphology. Molecular Neurodegeneration. 2007;**2**:12

[44] Zhang X, Tang N, Hadden TJ, Rishi AK. Akt, FoxO and regulation of apoptosis. Biochimica et Biophysica Acta, Molecular Cell Research. 2011;**1813**(11):1978-1986

[45] White MF. IRS2 integrates insulin/IGF1 signalling with metabolism, neurodegeneration and longevity. Diabetes, Obesity and Metabolism. 2014;**16**:4-15

[46] Bhaskar PT, Hay N. The two TORCs and Akt. Developmental Cell. 2007;**12**(4):487-502

[47] Kapahi P, Chen D, Rogers AN, Katewa SD, Li PWL, Thomas EL, et al. With TOR, less is more: A key role for the conserved nutrient-sensing TOR pathway in aging. Cell Metabolism. 2010;**11**(6):453-465

[48] O'Neill C. PI3-kinase/Akt/mTOR signaling: Impaired on/off switches in aging, cognitive decline and Alzheimer's disease. Experimental Gerontology. 2013;**48**(7):647-653

[49] López-Otín C, Blasco MA, Partridge L, Serrano M, Kroemer G. The hallmarks of aging. Cell. 2013;**153**(6):1194-1217

[50] Partridge L, Piper MDW, Mair W. Dietary restriction in *Drosophila*. Mechanisms of Ageing and Development. 2005;**126**:938-950

[51] Kenyon CJ. The genetics of ageing. Nature. 2010;**467**(7315):622-622

[52] Onken B, Driscoll M. Metformin induces a dietary restriction-like state and the oxidative stress response to extend C. elegans healthspan via AMPK, LKB1, and SKN-1. PLoS One. 2010;**5**(1):e8758

[53] Anisimov VN, Berstein LM, Popovich IG, Zabezhinski MA, Egormin PA, Piskunova TS, et al. If started early in life, metformin treatment increases life span and postpones tumors in female SHR mice. Aging. 2011;**3**(2):148-157

[54] Fontana L, Partridge L. Promoting health and longevity through diet: From model organisms to humans. Cell. 2015;**161**(1):106-118

[55] Amigo I, Menezes-Filho SL, Luevano-Martinez LA, Chausse B, Kowaltowski AJ. Caloric restriction increases brain mitochondrial calcium retention capacity and protects against excitotoxicity. Aging Cell. 2017;**16**(1):73-81

[56] Halicka HD, Zhao H, Li J, Traganos F, Zhang S, Lee M, et al. Genome protective effect of metformin as revealed by reduced level of constitutive DNA damage signaling. Aging (Albany NY). 2011;**3**(10):1028-1038

[57] Maiese K. mTOR: Driving apoptosis and autophagy for neurocardiac complications of diabetes mellitus. World Journal of Diabetes. 2015;**6**(2):217-224

[58] Haigis MC, Yankner BA. The aging stress response. Molecular Cell. 2010;**40**(2):333-344

[59] St-Pierre J, Drori S, Uldry M, Silvaggi JM, Rhee J, Jäger S, et al. Suppression of reactive oxygen species and neurodegeneration by the PGC-1 transcriptional coactivators. Cell. 2006;**127**(2):397-408

[60] Hipp MS, Park S-H, Hartl FU. Proteostasis impairment in protein-misfolding and aggregation diseases. Trends in Cell Biology. 2014;**24**(9):506-514

[61] Madabhushi R, Pan L, Tsai LH. DNA damage and its links to neurodegeneration. Neuron. 2014;**83**(2):266-282

[62] Fontana L, Meyer TE, Klein S, Holloszy JO. Long-term calorie restriction is highly effective in reducing the risk for atherosclerosis in humans. Proceedings of the National Academy of Sciences of the United States of America. 2004;**101**(17):6659-6663

[63] Meyer TE, Kovács SJ, Ehsani AA, Klein S, Holloszy JO, Fontana L. Long-term caloric restriction ameliorates the decline in diastolic function in humans. Journal of the American College of Cardiology. 2006;**47**(2):398-402

[64] Colman RJ, Anderson RM, Johnson SC, Kastman EK, Kosmatka KJ, Beasley TM, et al. Caloric restriction delays disease onset and mortalilty in rhesus monkeys. Science. 2009;**325**(5937):201-204

[65] Fontana L, Klein S, Holloszy JO. Effects of long-term calorie restriction and endurance exercise on glucose tolerance, insulin action, and adipokine production. Age (Omaha). 2010;**32**(1):97-108

[66] Redman LM, Smith SR, Burton JH, Martin CK, Il'yasova D, Ravussin E.

Metabolic slowing and reduced oxidative damage with sustained caloric restriction support the rate of living and oxidative damage theories of aging. Cell Metabolism. 2018;**27**(4):805, e4-815

[67] Il'yasova D, Fontana L, Bhapkar M, Pieper CF, Spasojevic I, Redman LM, et al. Effects of 2 years of caloric restriction on oxidative status assessed by urinary F2-isoprostanes: The CALERIE 2 randomized clinical trial. Aging Cell. 2018;**17**(2):e12719

[68] Fontana L, Villareal DT, Das SK, Smith SR, Meydani SN, Pittas AG, et al. Effects of 2 year calorie restriction on circulating levels of IGF-1, IGF-binding proteins and cortisol in nonobese men and women: A randomized clinical trial. Aging Cell. 2016;**15**(1):22-27

[69] Levine ME, Suarez JA, Brandhorst S, Balasubramanian P, Cheng CW, Madia F, et al. Low protein intake is associated with a major reduction in IGF-1, cancer, and overall mortality in the 65 and younger but not older population. Cell Metabolism. 2014;**19**(3):407-417

[70] Masters CL, Bateman R, Blennow K, Rowe CC, Sperling RA, Cummings JL. Alzheimer's disease. Nature Reviews. Disease Primers. 2015;**1**:15056

[71] Alzheimer's Disease International. World Alzheimer Report 2018— The State of the Art of Dementia Research: New Frontiers. 2018th ed. London: Alzheimer's Disease International; 2018. 48 p. Available from: https://www.alz.co.uk/research/WorldAlzheimerReport2018.pdf

[72] Golde TE, Eckman CB, Younkin SG. Biochemical detection of Abeta isoforms: Implications for pathogenesis, diagnosis, and treatment of Alzheimer's disease. Biochimica et Biophysica Acta. 2000;**1502**(1):172-187

[73] Yang Y, Song W. Molecular links between Alzheimer's disease and diabetes mellitus. Neuroscience. 2013;**250**:140-150

[74] Mittal K, Katare DP. Shared links between type 2 diabetes mellitus and Alzheimer's disease: A review. Diabetes and Metabolic Syndrome: Clinical Research & Reviews. 2016;**10**(2):S144-S149

[75] Chatterjee S, Mudher A. Alzheimer's disease and type 2 diabetes: A critical assessment of the shared pathological traits. Frontiers in Neuroscience. 2018;**12**:383

[76] Xu W, Caracciolo B, Wang H-X, Winblad B, Backman L, Qiu C, et al. Accelerated progression from mild cognitive impairment to dementia in people with diabetes. Diabetes. 2010;**59**(11):2928-2935

[77] Cheng G, Huang C, Deng H, Wang H. Diabetes as a risk factor for dementia and mild cognitive impairment: A meta-analysis of longitudinal studies. Internal Medicine Journal. 2012;**42**(5):484-491

[78] Sanz CM, Hanaire H, Vellas BJ, Sinclair AJ, Andrieu S. REAL.FR study group. Diabetes mellitus as a modulator of functional impairment and decline in Alzheimer's disease. The Real.FR cohort. Diabetic Medicine. 2012;**29**(4):541-548

[79] Silzer TK, Phillips NR. Etiology of type 2 diabetes and Alzheimer's disease: Exploring the mitochondria. Mitochondrion. 2018;**43**:16-24

[80] Lourenco MV, Ferreira ST, De Felice FG. Neuronal stress signaling and eIF2a phosphorylation as molecular links between Alzheimer's disease and diabetes. Progress in Neurobiology. 2015;**129**:37-57

[81] Ribe EM, Lovestone S. Insulin signalling in Alzheimer's disease and diabetes: From epidemiology to molecular links. Journal of Internal Medicine. 2016;**280**(5):430-442

[82] Zhang J, Chen C, Hua S, Liao H, Wang M, Xiong Y, et al. An updated meta-analysis of cohort studies: Diabetes and risk of Alzheimer's disease. Diabetes Research and Clinical Practice. 2017;**124**:41-47

[83] Steen E, Terry BM, Rivera EJ, Cannon JL, Neely TR, Tavares R, et al. Impaired insulin and insulin-like growth factor expression and signaling mechanisms in Alzheimer's disease—Is this type 3 diabetes? Journal of Alzheimer's Disease. 2005;**7**(1):63-80

[84] Caccamo A, Belfiore R, Oddo S. Genetically reducing mTOR signaling rescues central insulin dysregulation in a mouse model of Alzheimer's disease. Neurobiology of Aging. 2018;**68**:59-67

[85] Ali M, Bukhari SA, Ali M, Lee H-W. Upstream signalling of mTORC1 and its hyperactivation in type 2 diabetes (T2D). BMB Reports. 2017;**50**(12):601-609

[86] Tramutola A, Triplett JC, Di Domenico F, Niedowicz DM, Murphy MP, Coccia R, et al. Alteration of mTOR signaling occurs early in the progression of Alzheimer disease (AD): Analysis of brain from subjects with pre-clinical AD, amnestic mild cognitive impairment and late-stage AD. Journal of Neurochemistry. 2015;**133**(5):739-749

[87] Nelson TJ, Alkon DL. Insulin and cholesterol pathways in neuronal function, memory and neurodegeneration. Biochemical Society Transactions. 2005;**33**(5):1033

[88] Reddy VP, Zhu X, Perry G, Smith MA. Oxidative stress in diabetes and Alzheimer's disease. Journal of Alzheimer's Disease. 2009;**16**(4):763-774

[89] De Felice FG, Ferreira ST. Inflammation, defective insulin signaling, and mitochondrial dysfunction as common molecular denominators connecting type 2 diabetes to Alzheimer disease. Diabetes. 2014;**63**(7):2262-2272

[90] Olefsky JM, Glass CK. Macrophages, inflammation, and insulin resistance. Annual Review of Physiology. 2010;**72**(1):219-246

[91] Nikolajczyk BS, Jagannathan-Bogdan M, Shin H, Gyurko R. State of the union between metabolism and the immune system in type 2 diabetes. Genes and Immunity. 2011;**12**(4):239-250

[92] Stumvoll M, Goldstein BJ, Van Haeften TW. Type 2 diabetes: Principles of pathogenesis and therapy. Lancet. 2005;**365**(9467):1333-1346

[93] Lebrun P, Van Obberghen E. SOCS proteins causing trouble in insulin action. Acta Physiologica. 2008;**192**(1):29-36

[94] Sethi JK, Hotamisligil GS. The role of TNFα in adipocyte metabolism. Seminars in Cell & Developmental Biology. 1999;**10**(1):19-29

[95] Kohn LD, Wallace B, Schwartz F, McCall K. Is type 2 diabetes an autoimmune-inflammatory disorder of the innate immune system? Endocrinology. 2005;**146**(10):4189-4191

[96] Perry VH, Nicoll JAR, Holmes C. Microglia in neurodegenerative disease. Nature Reviews. Neurology. 2010;**6**(4):193-201

[97] Swardfager W, Lanctôt K, Rothenburg L, Wong A, Cappell J, Herrmann N. A meta-analysis of cytokines in Alzheimer's disease. Biological Psychiatry. 2010;**68**(10):930-941

[98] Schulingkamp RJ, Pagano TC, Hung D, Raffa RB. Insulin receptors

and insulin action in the brain: Review and clinical implications. Neuroscience and Biobehavioral Reviews. 2000;**24**(8):855-872

[99] Craft S. Insulin resistance and AD—Extending the translational path. Nature Reviews. Neurology. 2012;**8**(7):360-362

[100] Li L, Hölscher C. Common pathological processes in Alzheimer disease and type 2 diabetes: A review. Brain Research Reviews. 2007;**56**(2):384-402

[101] Praticò D, Clark CM, Liun F, Lee VY-M, Trojanowski JQ. Increase of brain oxidative stress in mild cognitive impairment: A possible predictor of Alzheimer disease. Archives of Neurology. 2002;**59**(6):972-976

[102] Migliore L, Fontana I, Trippi F, Colognato R, Coppedè F, Tognoni G, et al. Oxidative DNA damage in peripheral leukocytes of mild cognitive impairment and AD patients. Neurobiology of Aging. 2005;**26**(5):567-573

[103] Xavier DJ, Takahashi P, Evangelista AF, Foss-Freitas MC, Foss MC, Donadi EA, et al. Assessment of DNA damage and mRNA/miRNA transcriptional expression profiles in hyperglycemic versus non-hyperglycemic patients with type 2 diabetes mellitus. Mutation Research-Fundamental and Molecular Mechanisms of Mutagenesis. 2015;**776**:98-110

[104] Shackelford DA. DNA end joining activity is reduced in Alzheimer's disease. Neurobiology of Aging. 2006;**27**(4):596-605

[105] Leandro GS, Evangelista AF, Lobo RR, Xavier DJ, Moriguti JC, Sakamoto-Hojo ET. Changes in expression profiles revealed by transcriptomic analysis in peripheral blood mononuclear cells of Alzheimer's disease patients. Journal of Alzheimer's Disease. 2018;**1**:1-13

[106] Ataian Y, Krebs JE. Five repair pathways in one context: Chromatin modification during DNA repair. Biochemistry and Cell Biology. 2006;**84**(4):490-494

Section 2

Diabetes and the Brain

Chapter 4

Cognitive Dysfunction in Diabetes Mellitus

Faiz Ahmed Shaikh, K.C. Bhuvan, Thet Thet Htar, Manish Gupta and Yatinesh Kumari

Abstract

People with diabetes mellitus type 2 will have higher rate of cognitive impairment than people that do not. Besides that, the effect of diabetes on the normal mental functions is often disregarded. This may be due to a lack of signs and standard assessment technique to measure the cognitive function of the diabetes patient. Hyperglycaemia which is common in people with diabetes has been associated with an increase in the possibility of developing Alzheimer's disease and vascular dementia in the both general public and people with cognitive impairment. It has been estimated that an individual with diabetes mellitus is 1.5 times more likely to experience cognitive dysfunction and dementia than a normal healthy individual. Alleviation of microvascular complications and hypoglycaemia is the key in treatment of DM to prevent cognitive decline.

Keywords: diabetes, cognition, age, glucose impairment, HbA1c

1. Introduction

According to the International Diabetes Federation, diabetes is one of the largest global health emergencies of the twenty-first century and is the top 10 causes of death globally [1]. Diabetes mellitus (DM) is a disease in which the human body cannot produce sufficient amount of insulin and fails to respond to the hormone insulin that will result to the abnormal increase of glucose level in the blood circulation resulting in hyperglycaemia [2]. It is a complex metabolic disorder which can damage multiple organs in the human body [3]. DM affects or even burdens individual and communities with huge economic cost and leads to a decrease in overall productivity [4]. The complications of DM, especially type 2, can be enhanced by comorbidities such as hypertension, stroke, etc. [5]. Diabetes is the leading problem of kidney failure, lower-limb amputation and also blindness among adults [6]. In Malaysia, diabetes is one of the main public health problems and is closely related to avoidable and premature death [7].

The World Health Organization (WHO) divides the DM into two major categories which are insulin-dependent diabetes mellitus (IDDM) or type 1 diabetes mellitus and non-insulin-dependent diabetes mellitus (NIDDM) or type 2 diabetes mellitus [8]. Approximately 90% of all diabetes cases in both developed and developing countries are NIDDM and can be found mostly in people more than 30 years old [9]. In type 1 DM, the pancreas cannot produce insulin, and the body has to completely rely on the synthetic insulin to reduce the glucose in the blood.

Type 1 DM is common in children, teenager as well as young adult [10]. DM can lead to complications such as diabetic nephropathy, diabetic retinopathy, ischaemic heart disease and many more [11]. The number of people with type 2 DM is increasing in every country with 79% of people with DM living in low- and middle-income countries [12].

1.1 Global and Malaysian scenario of type 2 DM

Some 425 million people worldwide, or 8.8% of adults, are estimated to have diabetes [13]. About 79% lives in low- and middle-income countries. If these trends continue, by 2045, some 629 million people will have diabetes [13]. The estimated population of Malaysia in 2018 is 32.4 million [14]. There were almost 3.49 million cases of diabetes in Malaysia in 2017 [15]. The percentage of population aged 15–64 years old (working age) increases from 69.6% in 2017 to 69.7% in 2018. The percentage of 65 years and over (old age) population increases from 6.3 to 6.5% for the same period [14]. The number of deaths was divided into two groups of ages which are age between 30 and 69 years old as well as ages more than 70 years old. For example, the number of diabetes deaths for female ages more than 70 years old was 1260 people compared to 1070 for males [13].

2. Cognitive function

Cognitive function can be defined as mental process (cerebral activities) that lead to the gaining of knowledge which allows people to carry out their daily life activities [16]. Cognitive functions are mainly related to remembering, solving problems, making decision and understanding the language, problems or even issues like personal issues and health issues, focus, attention and others [2]. It also can be defined as memory which is tested by the stimuli either spoken or presented using another talking format or talking memory [17]. Moreover, it can be related to the large spectrum of cognitive capability among the middle- and old-aged group of people, which are having dementia as well as maintaining normal physiological function [18].

2.1 Relationship of cognitive function with type 2 DM

Cognitive impairment is a type of disorder which has not been studied and explored as the complications of DM. At the same time, the association of DM with cognition is well acknowledged. The meta-analysis shows small to moderate performance decline in persons with diabetes relative to nondiabetic controls in each domain examined. The motor function is largely affected, while attention/concentration is affected minimally [19]. Another study shows that people with type 2 DM will have higher rate of cognitive impairment than people that do not have DM [20]. Besides that, the effect of diabetes on the normal mental functions is often disregarded. This may be due to lack of signs and standard assessment technique to measure the cognitive function of the diabetes patient [21]. Hyperglycaemia which is common in people with diabetes has been associated with an increase in the possibility of developing Alzheimer's disease and vascular dementia in both the general public and people with cognitive impairment [22]. It has been estimated that an individual with DM is 1.5 times more likely to experience cognitive dysfunction and dementia than a normal healthy individual [23].

Elderly people who are more than 65-year-old will have more than 20% chances to be diagnosed with both DM and impaired cognitive function [24]. Type 2 DM has been associated with few cognitive impairments such as decreases in psychomotor speed, processing speed, visual retention, attention, concentration and many more. It is understood that more significantly hyperglycaemia, vascular disease, hypoglycaemia and insulin resistance affect cognitive decline, but the exact pathophysiological mechanisms not of cognitive decline in diabetes are unclear [3]. The causes of cognitive decline in diabetes may be the direct effect of the chronic hyperglycaemia on the brain regions, blood lipid, blood pressure, hypoglycaemia and others [25].

2.2 Duration of DM and cognitive impairment

Several studies have studied about the linkage of DM with cognitive decline in elderly population. A perspective (over 20 years) cohort study in the USA with mid-age (mean age 58) diabetic patient reported that DM in the midlife was related to a significant increase in cognitive impairment. This study included 13,351 black and white adults aged 48–67 years old, and their cognitive function was examined using three cognitive tests, which are the delayed-word-recall test (DWRT), the digit substitution test (DSST) of Wechsler Adult Intelligence Scale-Revised (WAIS-R) and the word fluency test (WFT). The study also reported that a patient with poorly controlled DM might have bigger cognitive disorder than well-controlled ones and longer duration of DM will have increased chances of late-life cognitive disorder [26].

A cross-sectional study was conducted on 57 patients having type 2 DM. The result shows that patients with type 2 DM had low grades in the cognitive testing and poor performance in different cognitive function tasks which include the verbal relations, visual reasoning, short-term memory test and many more. Cognitive function is impaired more with the untreated DM patient than the treated group [25]. Cognitive dysfunction is nonlinearly related to the duration of diabetes. However, cognitive decline is more prominent when the duration of DM is more than 5 years and presence of hypertension which further increases the risk of cognitive impairment [21]. The patients having diabetes showed poor performance in the tests of recent memory, repetition and attention, as compared to the control group and DM, and the people with long history of DM are more at risk of cognitive decline [27]. It is concluded that cognitive function of diabetes type 2 patients should frequently be tested. This is because the duration of disease can be related with the decrease in cognitive function. As duration increases, impairment also increases [28].

2.3 Influence of age and cognitive impairment

A prospective study is done to observe and determine the impact of DM on the cognitive function impairment in the oldest of the old participants. The study was conducted using prospective population method. They have chosen approximately 599 participants with the respond rate of 87% with the age ranges from 85 to 90 years old. The memory function test does not show any differences between both diabetic and nondiabetic participants. Cognitive function of diabetic participants is affected when the time and speed test has been conducted [29].

The results of another research show that diabetic patients more than 65 years old have higher chances to be associated with impaired cognitive function [24]. Besides that, one more study was conducted that is related to assessing the status of cognitive function in people that have DM. The chosen patients were assessed by using MMSE and 3MS (the modified mini-mental state examination). The scores for both assessments were 30 and 100, respectively. At the same time, the relationships of age, gender and duration of diabetes and HbA1c among the DM with 3MS will also be assessed. The results of this study were diabetic patients have lower

MMSE and 3MS than nondiabetic patients. This mean cognitive function will be reduced as the age increases and when having DM [30].

The uncontrolled DM which is one of the risk factors for cognitive impairment and dementia especially in Alzheimer patients. Therefore, controlling DM can reduce the possibility to get cognitive impairment and Alzheimer disease [5].

2.4 Association between duration of DM and age towards cognitive impairment

According to a homogenous cohort study on the community-dwelling women in 11 US states. This study focusses on women that live in the community which are on their own compared to living in nursing or old folk home. The result of this research was participants (women) with type 2 DM had lower mean score in all the tests conducted than women without DM. At the same time, when duration has been diagnosed with DM and insufficiency in pharmacological treatment, it can worsen or cause increment in cognitive impairment. One of the limitations for this research is self-reporting regarding diabetes diagnosis [31].

Meanwhile, another study was done regarding the cognitive impairment in diabetic patients with special references to age of onset, duration and also control of diabetes. The study was conducted in diabetic patients that came to the medicine inpatient and outpatient departments and diabetic clinic of SSKM Hospital, India. It is used to calculate the mean effect of sugar control after a 6-month period. The result of this study was cognitive impairment has a relationship with diabetes. The cognitive function that usually affected were recognition, fluency and immediate memory power of the patients. Control of DM can help in improving cognitive function of the patients. Other habits such as smoking, poor control of sugar intake as well as life style can enhance the effect of cognitive impairment [32].

A cross-sectional study was conducted which is related to prevalence and predictors of cognitive dysfunction in type 2 DM population of Punjab, India. The study involves 516 type 2 DM participants that attended the endocrinology outpatient department of the Government Medical College and Hospital, Patiala, Punjab, India. The result of this study shows that many of diabetic participants that are living in Punjab, India, remain undiagnosed with cognitive impairment during their life. Cognitive impairment in diabetic participants is independently influenced by duration of diabetes, age of the patients and other complications besides diabetes such as hypertension and others [33].

2.5 HbA1c control and cognitive decline

HbA1c is recommended to be used to identify the people at risk of developing diabetes as well as to diagnose diabetes. It is the most important biomarker for the management of blood glucose control in individuals with already diagnosed diabetes [34]. It is also a strong predictor for ensuing diabetes, because it incorporates the average blood glucose level over the last 2–3 months [35] and has better reliability than fasting or postprandial blood glucose test [36]. The cohort studies conducted in middle-aged populations show that the cognitive decline in people with diabetes is significantly faster than those with normal blood glucose levels [26, 37]. The study also reported that there is no significant difference in cognitive decline in people with prediabetes than in those with normal blood glucose levels [13]. On the contrary, the other study reported significantly faster cognitive decline among people with prediabetes than those with normal HbA1c levels [26]. The longitudinal study done reported significant longitudinal associations between HbA1c levels, diabetes status and long-term cognitive decline [38].

3. Cognitive deficits in patients with type 1 and type 2 DM

The cognitive domains that were negatively affected have been identified in patients with type 1 and type 2 DM with strong supporting data (**Table 1**).

The cognitive domains that were negatively affected have been identified in patients with type 1 and type 2 DM with less supporting data (**Table 2**).

3.1 Physiological pathways linking diabetes and cognition

The link between diabetes and cognitive impairment was first reported in 1922 [58]. The exact physiologic pathways linking the two conditions remain unclear. The hypothetical mechanisms include which is related to cerebrovascular complications, neuronal glucose processing and frequent episodes of hypoglycaemia [3, 59, 60]. The diabetic patients are more prone to develop comorbid cardiovascular disease, which is itself predictive of cognitive decline through cerebrovascular events and other pathways [61].

3.2 Treatment strategy

There are some complications of type 2 DM that affect the brain; it is believed that diabetes treatment may have beneficial effects on cognition. Three different trials reported that intensive glycaemic control alleviate microvascular complications but does not alleviate macrovascular complications in geriatric patients with long-duration of type 2 diabetes and high cardiovascular risk [62–64]. The intensive treatment of type 2 DM leads to hypoglycaemia which may contribute to cognitive decline and eliminate the benefits of intensive treatment [63, 65, 66]. Hypoglycaemia is more common in intensive glycaemic control than in standard glycaemic control [67].

Type 1 DM	Type 2 DM
Slowing of information processing [39–42]	Psychomotor speed [43]
Psychomotor efficiency [39, 40, 44]	Memory
Attention [42]	Working memory [45, 46]
Visuoconstruction [42]	Verbal memory [47]
	Immediate recall
	Delayed recall [31]
	Executive function [43, 45, 46]

Table 1.
Cognitive domains affected by type 1 and type 2 DM (with strong supporting data).

Type 1 DM	Type 2 DM
Memory [44]	Verbal fluency [43, 48]
Motor speed [41, 49–51]	Complex motor function [43]
Vocabulary [44, 52–54]	Processing speed [47]
General intelligence [53, 54]	Attention [55]
Visual perception	Depression [45, 56]
Motor strength [51]	
Executive function [49, 57]	

Table 2.
Cognitive domains affected by type 1 and type 2 DM (with less supporting data).

4. Conclusion

DM is an important risk factor along with other diabetic complications for cognitive decline, which leads to loss of independence and nonadherence to medication and results in high healthcare cost. It is still controversial how early the age of cognitive impairment is, although there is enough documented links between diabetes and cognitive function. The standard glycaemic control is better than intensive glycaemic control in the prevention of cognitive decline. The challenge for treatment is to maintain the cognitive function by reduction of hypoglycaemic events.

Conflict of interest

There is no conflict of interest among the authors.

Author details

Faiz Ahmed Shaikh[1,2], K.C. Bhuvan[1*], Thet Thet Htar[1], Manish Gupta[1,3] and Yatinesh Kumari[4]

1 School of Pharmacy, Monash University Malaysia, Bandar Sunway, Selangor, Malaysia

2 Clinical Pharmacy Unit, School of Pharmacy, Management and Science University, Selangor, Malaysia

3 Faculty of Pharmacy, DIT University, Dehradun, India

4 Jeffrey Cheah School of Medicine and Health Sciences, Monash University Malaysia, Bandar Sunway, Selangor, Malaysia

*Address all correspondence to: bhuvan.kc@monash.edu

References

[1] Atlas ID. Brussels, Belgium: International diabetes federation; 2013. International Diabetes Federation (IDF). 2017

[2] Tomar S. Impact of neurobiofeedback therapy on cognitive impairment among type-2 diabetes mellitus patients. Delhi Psychiatry Journal. 2012;**15**(2):287-293

[3] Kodl CT, Seaquist ER. Cognitive dysfunction and diabetes mellitus. Endocrine Reviews. 2008;**29**(4):494-511

[4] Mafauzy M, Hussein Z, Chan S. The status of diabetes control in Malaysia: Results of DiabCare 2008. The Medical Journal of Malaysia. 2011;**66**(3):175-181

[5] Rajeshkanna N, Valli S, Thuvaragah P. Relation between diabetes mellitus type 2 and cognitive impairment: A predictor of alzheimer's disease. International Journal of Medical Research & Health Sciences. 2014;**3**(4):903-910

[6] Control CfD, Prevention. National Diabetes Fact Sheet: National Estimates and General Information on Diabetes and Prediabetes in the United States, 2011. Atlanta, GA: US department of health and human services, centers for disease control and prevention; 2011;201(1)

[7] Feisul M, Azmi S. National Diabetes Registry Report, Volume 1, 2009-2012. Kuala Lumpur: Ministry of Health Malaysia. p. 2013

[8] Organization WH. Definition, diagnosis and classification of diabetes mellitus and its complications: Report of a WHO consultation. In: Part 1, Diagnosis and Classification of Diabetes Mellitus. Geneva: World health organization; 1999

[9] Shaw JE, Sicree RA, Zimmet PZ. Global estimates of the prevalence of diabetes for 2010 and 2030. Diabetes Research and Clinical Practice. 2010;**87**(1):4-14

[10] Chiang JL, Kirkman MS, Laffel LM, Peters AL. Type 1 diabetes through the life span: A position statement of the American diabetes association. Diabetes Care. 2014;**37**(7):2034-2054

[11] Mafauzy M. Diabetes control and complications in public hospitals in Malaysia. Medical Journal of Malaysia. 2006;**61**(4):477

[12] Whiting DR, Guariguata L, Weil C, Shaw J. IDF diabetes atlas: Global estimates of the prevalence of diabetes for 2011 and 2030. Diabetes Research and Clinical Practice. 2011;**94**(3):311-321

[13] Ogurtsova K, da Rocha Fernandes J, Huang Y, Linnenkamp U, Guariguata L, Cho N, et al. IDF diabetes atlas: Global estimates for the prevalence of diabetes for 2015 and 2040. Diabetes Research and Clinical Practice. 2017;**128**:40-50

[14] Malaysia DoS. Population and Housing Census of Malaysia. Putrajaya: Department of Statistics Malaysia; 2010

[15] Forces ID. International Diabetes Federation Diabetes Atlas. Brussels, Belgium: International Diabetes Federation; 2015

[16] Bandura A. Social cognitive theory: An agentic perspective. Annual Review of Psychology. 2001;**52**(1):1-26

[17] Cosway R, Strachan M, Dougall A, Frier B, Deary I. Cognitive function and information processing in type 2 diabetes. Diabetic Medicine. 2001;**18**(10):803-810

[18] Huppert FA, Gardener E, McWilliams B. Cognitive function. In: Retirement, Health and Relationships of the Older Population in England.

London, UK: The Institute for Fiscal Studies; 2004. pp. 217-242

[19] Palta P, Schneider AL, Biessels GJ, Touradji P, Hill-Briggs F. Magnitude of cognitive dysfunction in adults with type 2 diabetes: A meta-analysis of six cognitive domains and the most frequently reported neuropsychological tests within domains. Journal of the International Neuropsychological Society. 2014;**20**(3):278-291

[20] Cukierman T, Gerstein H, Williamson J. Cognitive decline and dementia in diabetes—Systematic overview of prospective observational studies. Diabetologia. 2005;**48**(12):2460-2469

[21] Hazari MAH, Reddy BR, Uzma N, Kumar BS. Cognitive impairment in type 2 diabetes mellitus. International Journal of Diabetes Mellitus. 2015;**3**(1):19-24

[22] Feinkohl I, Price JF, Strachan MW, Frier BM. The impact of diabetes on cognitive decline: Potential vascular, metabolic, and psychosocial risk factors. Alzheimer's Research & Therapy. 2015;**7**(1):46

[23] Cukierman-Yaffe T, Gerstein HC, Williamson JD, Lazar RM, Lovato L, Miller ME, et al. Relationship between baseline glycemic control and cognitive function in individuals with type 2 diabetes and other cardiovascular risk factors: The action to control cardiovascular risk in diabetes-memory in diabetes (ACCORD-MIND) trial. Diabetes Care. 2009;**32**(2):221-226

[24] Rodríguez-Sánchez E, Mora-Simón S, Patino-Alonso MC, Pérez-ArechaederraD,Recio-RodríguezJI, Gómez-Marcos MA, et al. Cognitive impairment and dependence of patients with diabetes older than 65 years old in an urban area (DERIVA study). BMC Geriatrics. 2016;**16**(1):33

[25] Hamed SA, Youssef A, Elserogy Y, Herdan O, Abd-Elaal R, Metwaly N, et al. Cognitive function in patients with type 2 diabetes mellitus: Relationship to stress hormone (cortisol). Journal of Neurology and Neuroscience. 2013;**4**:3

[26] Rawlings AM, Sharrett AR, Schneider AL, Coresh J, Albert M, Couper D, et al. Diabetes in midlife and cognitive change over 20 years: A cohort study. Annals of Internal Medicine. 2014;**161**(11):785-793

[27] Kalar MU, Mujeeb E, Pervez S, Lalani Z, Raza B, Batool A, et al. Assessment of cognitive status in type 2 diabetes. International Journal of Collaborative Research on Internal Medicine & Public Health. 2014;**6**(8):235

[28] Alencar RC, Cobas RA, Gomes MB. Assessment of cognitive status in patients with type 2 diabetes through the mini-mental status examination: A cross-sectional study. Diabetology and Metabolic Syndrome. 2010;**2**(1):10

[29] Van den Berg E, De Craen A, Biessels G, Gussekloo J, Westendorp R. The impact of diabetes mellitus on cognitive decline in the oldest of the old: A prospective population-based study. Diabetologia. 2006;**49**(9):2015-2023

[30] Shuba N. Assessment of the cognitive status in diabetes mellitus. Journal of Clinical and Diagnostic Research: JCDR. 2012;**6**(10):1658

[31] Grodstein F, Chen J, Wilson RS, Manson JE. Type 2 diabetes and cognitive function in community-dwelling elderly women. Diabetes Care. 2001;**24**(6):1060-1065

[32] Mukherjee P, Mazumdar S, Goswami S, Bhowmik J, Chakroborty S, Mukhopadhyay S, et al. Cognitive dysfunction in diabetic patients with special reference to age of

onset, duration and control of diabetes. Activitas Nervosa Superior. 2012;**54**(1-2):67-75

[33] Khullar S, Kaur G, Dhillon H, Sharma R, Mehta K, Singh M, et al. The prevalence and predictors of cognitive impairment in type 2 diabetic population of Punjab, India. Journal of Social Health and Diabetes. 2017;**5**(1):47

[34] American Diabetes Association. Diagnosis and classification of diabetes mellitus. Diabetes Care. 2010;**33**(Supplement 1):S62-S69

[35] Selvin E, Steffes MW, Zhu H, Matsushita K, Wagenknecht L, Pankow J, et al. Glycated hemoglobin, diabetes, and cardiovascular risk in nondiabetic adults. The New England Journal of Medicine. 2010;**362**(9):800-811

[36] Selvin E, Crainiceanu CM, Brancati FL, Coresh J. Short-term variability in measures of glycemia and implications for the classification of diabetes. Archives of Internal Medicine. 2007;**167**(14):1545-1551

[37] Tuligenga RH, Dugravot A, Tabák AG, Elbaz A, Brunner EJ, Kivimäki M, et al. Midlife type 2 diabetes and poor glycaemic control as risk factors for cognitive decline in early old age: A post-hoc analysis of the Whitehall II cohort study. The Lancet Diabetes & Endocrinology. 2014;**2**(3):228-235

[38] Zheng F, Yan L, Yang Z, Zhong B, Xie W. HbA 1c, diabetes and cognitive decline: The english longitudinal study of ageing. Diabetologia. 2018;**61**(4):839-848

[39] Brands AM, Kessels RP, Hoogma RP, Henselmans JM, van der Beek Boter JW, Kappelle LJ, et al. Cognitive performance, psychological well-being, and brain magnetic resonance imaging in older patients with type 1 diabetes. Diabetes. 2006;**55**(6):1800-1806

[40] Ryan CM, Geckle MO, Orchard TJ. Cognitive efficiency declines over time in adults with type 1 diabetes: Effects of micro- and macrovascular complications. Diabetologia. 2003;**46**(7):940-948

[41] Ryan CM, Williams TM, Finegold DN, Orchard TJ. Cognitive dysfunction in adults with type 1 (insulin-dependent) diabetes mellitus of long duration: Effects of recurrent hypoglycaemia and other chronic complications. Diabetologia. 1993;**36**(4):329-334

[42] Wessels AM, Rombouts SA, Remijnse PL, Boom Y, Scheltens P, Barkhof F, et al. Cognitive performance in type 1 diabetes patients is associated with cerebral white matter volume. Diabetologia. 2007;**50**(8):1763-1769

[43] Reaven GM, Thompson LW, Nahum D, Haskins E. Relationship between hyperglycemia and cognitive function in older NIDDM patients. Diabetes Care. 1990;**13**(1):16-21

[44] Weinger K, Jacobson AM, Musen G, Lyoo IK, Ryan CM, Jimerson DC, et al. The effects of type 1 diabetes on cerebral white matter. Diabetologia. 2008;**51**(3):417-425

[45] Munshi M, Grande L, Hayes M, Ayres D, Suhl E, Capelson R, et al. Cognitive dysfunction is associated with poor diabetes control in older adults. Diabetes Care. 2006;**29**(8):1794-1799

[46] Perlmuter LC, Hakami MK, Hodgson-Harrington C, Ginsberg J, Katz J, Singer DE, et al. Decreased cognitive function in aging non-insulin-dependent diabetic patients. The American Journal of Medicine. 1984 Dec 1;**77**(6):1043-1048

[47] Messier C. Impact of impaired glucose tolerance and type 2 diabetes on cognitive aging. Neurobiology of Aging. 2005;**26**(1):26-30

[48] Kanaya AM, Barrett-Connor E, Gildengorin G, Yaffe K. Change in cognitive function by glucose tolerance status in older adults: A 4-year prospective study of the Rancho Bernardo study cohort. Archives of Internal Medicine. 2004;**164**(12):1327-1333

[49] Hershey T, Bhargava N, Sadler M, White NH, Craft S. Conventional versus intensive diabetes therapy in children with type 1 diabetes: Effects on memory and motor speed. Diabetes Care. 1999;**22**(8):1318-1324

[50] Ryan CM. Neurobehavioral complications of type I diabetes: Examination of possible risk factors. Diabetes Care. 1988;**11**(1):86-93

[51] Skenazy JA, Bigler ED. Neuropsychological findings in diabetes mellitus. Journal of Clinical Psychology. 1984;**40**(1):246-258

[52] Hershey T, Craft S, Bhargava N, White NH. Memory and insulin dependent diabetes mellitus (IDDM): Effects of childhood onset and severe hypoglycemia. Journal of the International Neuropsychological Society. 1997;**3**(6):509-520

[53] Northam EA, Anderson PJ, Werther GA, Warne GL, Adler RG, Andrewes D. Neuropsychological complications of IDDM in children 2 years after disease onset. Diabetes Care. 1998;**21**(3):379-384

[54] Schoenle EJ, Schoenle D, Molinari L, Largo RH. Impaired intellectual development in children with type I diabetes: Association with HbA1 c, age at diagnosis and sex. Diabetologia. 2002;**45**(1):108-114

[55] Fontbonne A, Berr C, Ducimetière P, Alpérovitch A. Changes in cognitive abilities over a 4-year period are unfavorably affected in elderly diabetic subjects: Results of the epidemiology of vascular aging study. Diabetes Care. 2001;**24**(2):366-370

[56] Bruce DG, Casey GP, Grange V, Clarnette RC, Almeida OP, Foster JK, et al. Cognitive impairment, physical disability and depressive symptoms in older diabetic patients: The fremantle cognition in diabetes study. Diabetes Research and Clinical Practice. 2003;**61**(1):59-67

[57] Northam EA, Anderson PJ, Jacobs R, Hughes M, Warne GL, Werther GA. Neuropsychological profiles of children with type 1 diabetes 6 years after disease onset. Diabetes Care. 2001;**24**(9):1541-1546

[58] Miles WR, Root HF. Psychologic tests applied to diabetic patients. Archives of Internal Medicine. 1922;**30**(6):767-777

[59] Awad N, Gagnon M, Messier C. The relationship between impaired glucose tolerance, type 2 diabetes, and cognitive function. Journal of Clinical and Experimental Neuropsychology. 2004;**26**(8):1044-1080

[60] Stolk RP, Breteler MM, Ott A, Pols HA, Lamberts SW, Grobbee DE, et al. Insulin and cognitive function in an elderly population: The Rotterdam study. Diabetes Care. 1997;**20**(5):792-795

[61] Leritz EC, McGlinchey RE, Kellison I, Rudolph JL, Milberg WP. Cardiovascular disease risk factors and cognition in the elderly. Current Cardiovascular Risk Reports. 2011;**5**(5):407

[62] Action to Control Cardiovascular Risk in Diabetes Study Group. Effects of intensive glucose lowering in type 2 diabetes. The New England Journal of Medicine. 2008;**358**(24):2545-2559

[63] ADVANCE Collaborative Group. Intensive blood glucose control and

vascular outcomes in patients with type 2 diabetes. The New England Journal of Medicine. 2008;**358**(24):2560-2572

[64] Turnbull FM, Abraira C, Anderson RJ, et al. Diabetologia. 2009;**52**:2288. Available from: https://doi.org/10.1007/s00125-009-1470-0

[65] Launer LJ, Miller ME, Williamson JD, Lazar RM, Gerstein HC, Murray AM, et al. Effects of intensive glucose lowering on brain structure and function in people with type 2 diabetes (ACCORD MIND): A randomised open-label substudy. The Lancet Neurology. 2011;**10**(11):969-977

[66] Cukierman-Yaffe T, Bosch J, Diaz R, Dyal L, Hancu N, Hildebrandt P, et al. Effects of basal insulin glargine and omega-3 fatty acid on cognitive decline and probable cognitive impairment in people with dysglycaemia: A substudy of the ORIGIN trial. The Lancet Diabetes & Endocrinology. 2014;**2**:562-572

[67] Chatterjee S, Sharma A, Lichstein E, Mukherjee D. Intensive glucose control in diabetics with an acute myocardial infarction does not improve mortality and increases risk of hypoglycemia-a meta-regression analysis. Current Vascular Pharmacology. 2013;**11**(1):100-104

Section 3

Management of Type 2 Diabetes

Chapter 5

SGLT2 Inhibitors Therapy in Type 2 Diabetes Mellitus

Maswood M. Ahmad, Imad Addin Brema and Mussa H. Almalki

Abstract

Type 2 diabetes mellitus (T2DM) is a chronic progressive disease characterized by chronic hyperglycemia and increased risk of cardiovascular disease (CVD). It results from multiple defects that lead to defective regulation of the blood glucose and requires continuous medical care with multifactorial risk-reduction strategies beyond glycemic control. Multiple groups of drugs have been approved in the past decades that work through different mechanisms. Apart from their limited efficacy in reducing cardiovascular outcome, most of them are neutral, and some may even increase mortality from CVDs such as rosiglitazone. The kidney has an important role in glucose regulation that was only recently targeted for drug development. Sodium-glucose cotransporter 2 inhibitors (SGLT2-I) are a new class of oral anti-hyperglycemic (OAH) agents that mainly act by preventing the reabsorption of filtered glucose by renal convoluted tubules. By their insulin-independent unique mechanism of action, SGLT2-I result in treating hyperglycemia while avoiding hypoglycemia, promote weight loss, reduce blood pressure, and, more importantly, decrease the risk of major adverse cardiovascular events (MACE). Therefore, SGLT2-I address fundamental aspects of the unmet needs of T2DM management that most of the other OAH failed to resolve. The main side effects of SGLT2-I are slight increase in the incidence of genital mycotic infections (GMI) and euglycemic ketoacidosis (EKA) along with increased risk of lower limb amputations, which has been reported with some but not all agents of this class.

Keywords: type 2 diabetes mellitus, SGLT2 inhibitors, hyperglycemia, cardiovascular disease, mycotic infections, euglycemic ketoacidosis

1. Introduction

T2DM is a chronic progressive metabolic disease characterized by chronic hyperglycemia and increased risk of CVDs that result from defective regulation of the blood glucose and requires continuous medical care with multifactorial risk-reduction strategies beyond glycemic control [1].

The magnitude of the problem can be assessed from the report of International Diabetes Federation (IDF) Atlas, where it was estimated that in 2017 there were 451 million people (age 18–99 years) with diabetes mellitus (DM) worldwide and that almost half of all people (49.7%) living with DM are undiagnosed [2]. More alarmingly, the projected figures for the prevalence of DM according to the same IDF report are expected to increase to 693 million by year 2045. In addition, there

IntechOpen

was an estimated 374 million people with impaired glucose tolerance (IGT), and in 2017 sadly, approximately 5 million deaths worldwide were attributable to DM. The global healthcare expenditure on people with DM was estimated to be USD 850 billion in 2017 [2]. Therefore, it is obvious that T2DM comes with a huge burden of morbidity and mortality and this is mainly due to the development of diabetes-specific microvascular complications and accelerated atherosclerotic macrovascular disease [3, 4].

T2DM is the seventh leading cause of death in the United States, and the estimate of the World Health Organization that T2DM-related mortality is expected to double in number by year 2030 if not treated properly further raises the alarm [5].

Improving glycemic control in people with DM not only substantially reduces their risk of microvascular complications and CVDs but also ameliorates the metabolic dysfunctions that contribute to the progressive nature and course of the disease. Evidence from United Kingdom Prospective Diabetes Study (UKPDS) showed that 1% reduction in glycosylated hemoglobin (HbA1C) was associated with relative risk reduction of 14% in fatal and nonfatal myocardial infarctions, 12% in fatal and nonfatal stroke, and 16% in heart failure [6].

While intensive glycemic control has been shown to substantially reduce the risk of microvascular complications, its value in reducing macrovascular complications that was previously reported 20 years after the end of UKPDS has recently been put in doubt after the ACCORD and ADVANCE Trials, which either showed increased risk of death or no benefit [7–9].

The UKPDS was the first study to show unequivocally that in patients with newly diagnosed T2DM, lowering blood glucose with intensive therapy to a median HbA1C of 7.0% was associated with 25% reduction in the rate of microvascular complications [7].

Moreover, after 10 years of follow-up post UKPDS, the benefits continued with regard to reduction in microvascular complication, and the reduction in macrovascular events was clearer [10].

Notable are the results of ACCORD, ADVANCE, and the Veterans Affairs Diabetes Trial (VADT) studies in patients with advanced T2DM, and either known CVD or multiple CVD risk factors showed that lowering blood glucose (HbA1C levels 6.4–6.9%) delayed the onset or slowed the progression of microvascular complications, but there was no significant reduction in CVD outcomes [8, 9, 11]. On the other hand, the ACCORD study suggests that less intensive therapy may be more appropriate in patients with T2DM and high risk of CVDs because intensive therapy to target HbA1C levels (6.4–7.5) was associated with a 22% increased risk of all-cause mortality [9].

Based on what we have learned from these studies, the American Diabetes Association and the European Association for the Study of Diabetes guideline suggest reducing HbA1C levels to around 7%, but in younger patients with short duration of diabetes and no significant heart diseases, HbA1C levels can be reduced to less than 6.5%. In older patients and those with advanced CVD and limited life expectancy, less stringent HbA1C levels around 8% may be appropriate [3].

Hypoglycemia, weight gain, and progressive beta-cell failure are the major limiting factors for intensive glycemic control approach and in achieving the proposed HbA1C goals [12].

The efficacy of the available OAHs and their effectiveness in the management of T2DM were reported in 2013 according to which and despite availability of several therapeutic options, 33–49% of patients fail to meet the targets for control of glycemia, blood pressure, or cholesterol and only a minority, around 14%, were able to meet targets for all three measures [13].

Apart from the limited efficacy of some OAHs in reducing CV risk, most of these agents are neutral when it comes to CVD risk reduction and some may even increase mortality from CVDs.

Therefore, for some time, T2DM unmet needs remained unresolved, and the need for innovation continued. For some experts in the field, it was suggested that newer OAHs should be so unique in their properties, namely, addressing the unmet needs and filling the gaps of the available OAHs such as weight gain, hypoglycemia, and CV safety to pass the test of FDA approval after the rosiglitazone story which was withdrawn from the market in 2008 because of its association with increased risk of CVDs [14]. Following rosiglitazone incident, the FDA mandated cardiovascular outcome trials on all newer OAH agents [15].

T2DM treatment requires individualized management with consideration of a number of patient factors. These include the degree of HbA1c reduction needed, risk of hypoglycemia, the side effect profile of medications, comorbid medical conditions, and the ability of patients to adhere to the medication regimen along with their preferences. Development of novel drugs with newer and complimentary mechanisms of action is needed to address the unwanted side effects and limitations of most of the old OAH agents, namely, the risk of hypoglycemia, weight gain, durability, and CV safety profile. Availability of newer medications with such profiles will simplify therapy and enhance patient adherence, especially in this era of increasing obesity.

Among newer classes of drugs, SGLT2-I hold great promise, and several agents from this group have already been approved by the US FDA and elsewhere for treatment of T2DM. They have a novel therapeutic mechanism of action when compared with other drugs available for T2DM management. The main site of action of SGLT2 inhibitors is in kidneys—a site which plays a major role in glucose homeostasis and has never been explored before.

2. Glucose homeostasis

Glucose is an essential and principal fuel source for cellular metabolism in the human body and is the main energy resource for the central nervous system, muscles, and fat—and insulin plays a key role in its effective utilization. The glucose homeostasis is rapidly adjusted in response to physiological changes such as food intake, exercise, and acute stress, and its blood level is adjusted by control of absorption of glucose, its metabolism in the liver, its excretion by kidneys, and uptake into muscles and adipose tissue. Functions of various proteins associated with regulation of glucose metabolism and homoeostasis get affected by diseases such as DM and hepatic disorders [16].

2.1 Handling of glucose in the intestine

After ingestion of carbohydrate-rich diet, blood glucose is regulated in response to the increase in glucose concentration in the intestinal lumen and in response to the increase in blood glucose level. The increase in glucose levels in the lumen of the small intestine provides a signal for the upregulation of intestinal glucose absorption [17] and leads to secretion of gut hormones such as glucose-dependent insulinotropic peptide (GIP) and glucagon-like peptide-1 (GLP-1), which increase the glucose-dependent stimulation of insulin secretion from the pancreatic β-cells and also influence appetite [18]. Insulin reduces glucagon secretion by acting on pancreatic alpha cells and also reduces blood glucose level by increasing glucose uptake in fat and muscle cells and changing glucose metabolism in the liver [1].

2.2 Glucose transport across plasma membrane

Being a highly polar molecule, glucose is unable to cross the lipid bilayer of the plasma membrane of all living cells; therefore, transport proteins within the cell membrane are required to facilitate glucose transport from the extracellular to the intracellular space.

Two distinct groups of glucose transporters belonging to solute carrier gene series (SLC) containing more than 50 transporter families have been described [19]. The first one is facilitated glucose transporters (GLUT) which is encoded by the SLC2 family of transporters GLUT1–4 and GLUT6–12, which help in passive transportation of glucose from the extracellular to the intracellular space along its chemical gradient without consuming any energy and equilibrate glucose concentration on both sides of membrane. The other one is sodium-glucose cotransporters (SGLTs) which are encoded by SLC5 family of transporters SGLT1–6 which actively transport glucose across plasma membranes against its concentration gradient. This process requires energy which is provided by simultaneous coupled transportation of sodium along its concentration gradient [19]. In this way, SGLTs help in concentrating glucose inside the cells.

The two principal sites of action of SGLTs are the intestine and kidney where they mediate glucose transportation across the intestinal lumen and the epithelial cells in the proximal renal tubules, respectively [20].

2.3 Handling of glucose by the kidney

The kidney plays an important role in glucose homeostasis by the process of filtration and reabsorption. Renal glomeruli filter approximately 180 liters of plasma daily which translates into filtration of approximately 180 g of glucose. In normal healthy subjects, all of this glucose is reabsorbed completely so that virtually no glucose is excreted in urine. Around 90% of the filtered renal glucose is reabsorbed in early part (S1) of proximal convoluted tubules by low-affinity high-capacity SGLT2. High-affinity low-capacity SGLT1 in distal straight segment (S3) of the proximal tubules reabsorbs the remaining 10% of the filtered renal glucose [21].

This process of glucose reabsorption is achieved by active Na^+ removal at basolateral surface by the Na^+/K^+-ATPase which generates the electrochemical driving force for apical glucose entry via Na^+-driven SGLTs. Reabsorbed glucose exits from the basolateral surface of the cells along its concentration gradient primarily via GLUT2 and reenters the bloodstream [21].

When blood glucose level exceeds 200 mg/dL, the excess glucose starts appearing in urine as renal transport maximum (T_m) of glucose is reached. The blood glucose level at which T_m is reached is called threshold and is around 300 mg/dL in healthy nondiabetic individuals, but glucose starts appearing in urine at around 200 mg/dL due to heterogeneity of individual nephrons in their T_m property and mismatch between glomerular filtration and tubular reabsorption of glucose. This safety valve-like action prevents extreme hyperglycemia [22].

The T_m of the proximal tubules on average is around 375 mg/minute although it shows inter-individual variations. The filtered glucose load is directly proportional to blood glucose concentration. In normal nondiabetic individuals, the filtered glucose load is less than 375 mg/minute; therefore, the entire amount is reabsorbed, and their urine is free of any glucose. This process has survival benefits as it allows the kidneys to conserve glucose and can be viewed as an adaptive mechanism.
In patients with T2DM, the filtered load may exceed 375 mg/minute; therefore, the T_m is exceeded, and all glucose in excess of the T_m spills over in urine [21]. In T2DM subjects, this adaptive mechanism becomes maladaptive. The increased expression of SGLT1/SGLT2 occurring in DM subjects results in increased renal

glucose reabsorption which ultimately leads to maintenance of a state of persistent hyperglycemia [23, 24]. The tubular growth leads to increased T_m for glucose which further exacerbates hyperglycemia [22].

Based upon these facts, the contribution of the kidney in development and maintenance of state of hyperglycemia in T2DM is quite evident. Therefore, SGLT2-I provide a pathophysiologically rational and novel approach to its treatment.

3. Clinical effects of mutations in SGLT1 and SGLT2

Autosomal recessive mutations in SGLT1 lead to a disorder called glucose galactose malabsorption (GGM). SGLT1 becomes nonfunctional, and infants with GGM develop severe watery diarrhea, dehydration, and metabolic acidosis that cease on diet free of glucose, galactose, and lactose [25].

In 1927, the first case of familial renal glycosuria was reported, in which a mutation in gene for SGLT2 resulted in loss of glucose in urine ranging from 1 to 150 g per 1.73 m^2 body surface areas per day. Almost 50 mutations have been identified so far leading to this condition which is characterized by urinary glucose excretion in the presence of normal plasma glucose levels and an absence of signs of general renal tubular dysfunction. Patients have normal oral glucose tolerance test and usually present with osmotic symptoms without any serious complications [26, 27]. The condition is not associated with any change in intravascular volume, serum glucose levels, or renal or bladder dysfunctions. These patients do not show higher incidence of kidney disease, DM, or urinary tract infections although those affected with severe forms of the disease may demonstrate activation of renin-angiotensin-aldosterone axis as indirect evidence of volume contraction [20, 26, 27].

These observations further strengthen the belief that SGLT2-I could potentially be developed as safe OAH.

4. Sodium-glucose cotransporters

So far, six different SGLTs have been described; however, apart from SGLT1 and SGLT2 which are well characterized, little is known about the function and clinical significance of the others [20]. Both SGLT1 and SGLT2 are large-membrane proteins consisting of 670 amino acids, and each has 14 transmembrane helical domains. The homology between SGLT1 and SGLT2 is around 58% (**Table 1**) [20].

Transporter	Gene	Substrate	Distribution and localization
SGLT1 (SLC5A1)	22q12.3	Glucose, galactose	Intestine, trachea, kidney, heart, brain, testis, prostate
SGLT2 (SLC5A2)	16p12.p11	Glucose	Kidney, brain, liver, thyroid, heart, muscle
SGLT3 (SLC5A4)	21q22.12	Glucose	Intestine, testis, uterus, lung, brain, thyroid
SGLT4 (SLC5A9)	1p32	Glucose, mannose	Intestine, kidney, liver, brain, lung, trachea, uterus, pancreas
SGLT5 (SLC5A10)	17p11.2	Glucose, galactose	Renal cortex
SGLT6 (SLC5A11)	16p12.1	D-chiro-inositol	Spinal cord, kidney, brain

Table 1.
Genes, substrates, and distributions of SGLT [28].

4.1 Sodium-glucose cotransporter 1 (SGLT1)

4.1.1 Locations of SGLT1

Studies have classically localized SGLT1 to the small intestine and the kidney where their pathophysiological roles are known in details [28].

Various other body organs such as the heart, lung, trachea, liver, skeletal muscle, gall bladder, rectum, colon, brain, blood vessels, breast, uterus, testis, and pancreatic alpha cells have shown mRNA level expression of SGLT1 [28–33].

4.1.2 Functional properties of SGLT1

SGLT1 transports one molecule of glucose or galactose together with two sodium ions. This stoichiometric ratio of 1:2 enables to raise the intracellular glucose level orders of magnitude above the corresponding extracellular concentration. The apparent Michaelis-Menten Km values for glucose and galactose at physiological extracellular sodium concentration and membrane potential are 0.5 and 1.0 mM, respectively. It has high affinity for both glucose and galactose but has a lower transport capacity (T_{max} = 2 nmol/mg protein per minute) [28, 34].

4.1.3 Physiological functions of SGLT1

SGLT1 is highly expressed in the small intestine and is located in the brush border membrane (BBM) of the enterocytes and in endocrine cells of gut and the K- and L-cells which secrete GIP and GLP-1/GLP-2, respectively. SGLT1-mediated translocation of glucose is the rate-limiting step for small intestinal glucose absorption [17, 28, 29]. Absorbed glucose in the enterocytes is released across the basolateral membrane and enters blood circulation via GLUT2. During bacterial infection, SGLT1 protects the small intestine from lipopolysaccharide-induced inflammation because of high luminal glucose concentrations [35].

In the kidney, SGLT1 is located at BBM of S3 segment of renal tubules and is responsible for the first and rate-limiting step in reabsorption of glucose which escaped SGLT2-mediated reabsorption in S1 and S2 segments. In normal healthy adults, it only absorbs around 10% of the filtered glucose load, but in DM patients with uncontrolled hyperglycemia, the fraction of SGLT1-mediated renal glucose absorption increases significantly. Similarly, in patients on SGLT2-I therapy, the fraction increases to around 50–70% [17, 28, 29]. SGLT1 may play a protective role during treatment with nephrotoxic drugs such as cisplatin [36].

SGLT1 mRNA has been detected in the frontal cortex, hypothalamus, and Purkinje cells of cerebellum and hippocampus in brains of human, rabbit, and rat [33, 37, 38]. It is mainly localized in the luminal membrane of the endothelial cells, and its location and functional activity suggests a pivotal role in securing energy supply to neurons during conditions of increased energy and glucose demand such as hypoxia and/or hypoglycemia. SGLT1-mediated neuronal glucose uptake is involved in glucose-induced neurotoxicity during ischemic stroke [39].

SGLT1 is located at the myocyte sarcolemma and in small blood vessels of the heart [29, 32]. SGLT1-mediated glucose uptake is of clinical significance as it leads to ATP generation by glycolysis during myocardial ischemia and/or hypoglycemia [40]. At the same time, it may increase toxic effects that are mediated by generation of reactive oxygen species (ROS) during hyperglycemia [41].

SGLTI1 mRNA has been detected in the lung, trachea, and bronchi, and its protein has been localized to alveolar type 2 cells and to the luminal membrane of bronchiolar Clara cells by immunohistochemistry [30, 31]. SGLT1-mediated glucose absorption contributes to fluid absorption and may provide energy for surfactant production in alveolar type 2 cells as well as for mucin and surfactants in Clara cells [42].

Similarly, the human gall bladder and liver have shown the presence of SGLT1 mRNA [29, 30]. Its expression at mRNA and protein level has been demonstrated in human pancreatic alpha cells; however, little is known about its functional role [30, 31]. SGLT1 has also been expressed in activated T-lymphocytes of mice where it may have a possible role in immune reactions [43].

4.1.4 Regulation of SGLT1 expression

The complex process of regulation of activity and expression of SGLT1 occurs in a tissue-specific manner. In the small intestine, upregulation of SGLT1 expression occurs in response to high-salt and/or high-glucose diet through transcriptional regulation which is also responsible for the circadian periodicity of SGLT1 expression [44, 45]. Its expression gets upregulated in the small intestine in diabetics [46] and in response to bacterial infections [35], while downregulation of SGLT1 expression occurs during chronic intestinal inflammation [47].

4.2 Sodium-glucose cotransporter 2 (SGLT2)

4.2.1 Locations of SGLT2

In humans, SGLT2 is strongly expressed in the kidney where it has been localized to the brush border membrane of the S1 and S2 segment of the proximal tubules. On the other hand, SGLT1 has been localized to the brush border membrane of the S3 segment of proximal convoluted tubules of the kidney [28–30, 48].

Proteins and mRNA of SGLT2 have also been found in alpha cells of the pancreas [31]. In addition to the kidney and pancreas, small amount of SGLT2 mRNA have been identified in the testis, liver, lung, and cerebellum [21, 28–30, 48].

4.2.2 Functional properties

SGLT2 is highly selective for glucose over galactose. It has low affinity for glucose with Km = 2 mM but with high transport capacity with T_{max} = 10 nmol/mg protein per minute and operates with a 1:1 stoichiometry of sodium and glucose. The apparent Michaelis-Menten Km values for glucose and sodium in human SGLT2 are 5 and 25 mM, respectively [28].

4.2.3 Physiological functions of SGLT2

4.2.3.1 Functions of SGLT2 in the kidney

Details of the physiological functions of SGLT2 in the kidney have already been mentioned earlier in Section 2.3.

In T2DM, SGLT2-mediated reabsorption of glucose and sodium is increased and can be considered physiologically maladaptive as it prevents an increase in urinary glucose excretion at high blood glucose levels. The increase in proximal tubular sodium reabsorption leads to fall in the distal tubular sodium and chloride concentrations which result in glomerular hyperfiltration [49] and plays a central role in the development of diabetic nephropathy [50].

The triad of hyperglycemia, elevated GFR, and the increased proximal tubular glucose reabsorption altogether leads to increase in kidney size and volume which is combined with glomerular hypertrophy, enlarged proximal tubules, inflammation, and interstitial fibrosis. These hyperglycemia-induced alterations lead to micro- and macroalbuminuria which culminate into renal failure [49].

4.2.3.2 Functions of SGLT2 in pancreatic alpha cells

During fasting when blood glucose level is low, several counter-regulatory responses are generated to increase and maintain blood glucose within normal range. Pancreatic alpha cells secrete glucagon which stimulates glycogenolysis and gluconeogenesis in the liver. Conversely, glucagon secretion is inhibited when blood glucose level increases after taking food [51]. Inhibition of glucagon secretion is mediated by paracrine effect of insulin and direct glucose-mediated regulation of glucagon secretion. In alpha cells, SGLT2-mediated glucose uptake is a critical step involved in direct regulation of glucagon secretion [31].

The expression of SGLT2 at mRNA level increases in alpha cells in obesity and prediabetes. Once T2DM develops, the glucotoxicity leads to decrease in its expression. The glucagon secretion blockage which normally occurs at high plasma glucose levels gets blunted due to downregulation of SGLT2 causing enhanced endogenous glucose production in the liver which further aggravates hyperglycemia [31].

4.2.4 Regulation of SGLT2

SGLT2 gene is located at chromosome 16 p11.2 and is expressed primarily in renal cortex. Various transcription factors are involved in regulation of SGLT2 such as SP-1, HNF1-alpha, and HNF4A, and their binding sites have been identified on SGLT2 promoter region [28].

High-sodium intake promotes urinary sodium and glucose excretion by increasing plasma adiponectin level through stimulation of peroxisome proliferator-activated receptor delta in adipose tissue. The enhanced adiponectin downregulates SGLT2 leading to reduced reabsorption of sodium and glucose. Due to hyperglycemia, this mechanism gets dampened in DM. Binding of SP-1 and HNF1-alpha at the promoter site is involved in this regulation [52], while HNF4A participates in glucose-dependent regulation of SGLT2 in alpha cells of the pancreas [31].

Activation of transcription factor NFκB (nuclear factor kappa-light-chain-enhancer of activated B cells) downregulates transcription of SGLT2 in the presence of hyperglycemia due to increase in ROS [53]. Sympathetic innervation has been found to be involved in transcriptional upregulation of SGLT2 in the kidney [54].

Posttranscriptional regulation of SGLT2 is yet to be understood well. Recently, it was found that the 17 kDa protein membrane-associated protein 17 (MAP17) upregulates functional activity of SGLT2 in the plasma membrane [55].

5. Development of SGLT inhibitors

Given the findings discussed in the above sections and considering the physiological functions of SGLT1 and SGLT2, it was an obvious idea to use SGLT1 and SGLT2 inhibitors as OAHs. Targeting hyperglycemia by inhibiting intestinal and renal glucose reabsorption appeared to be a novel therapeutic strategy.

Phlorizin was discovered around 150 years ago, which is a chemical found in the root bark, leaves, shoots, and fruit of the apple tree, and soon thereafter it was found to increase renal glucose excretion in healthy human beings. Phlorizin is a naturally occurring competitive nonselective inhibitor of SGLT1 and SGLT2.

In 1987, it was reported that subcutaneous phlorizin administration normalized plasma glucose profiles in insulin-resistant diabetic rats along with improving insulin sensitivity [56].

However, due to poor water solubility and poor oral bioavailability as it is metabolized to phloretin by glucosidase in gut and unselective SGLT1 and SGLT2 inhibition, phlorizin was not an ideal therapeutic agent. It has low selectivity for SGLT2 compared to SGLT1.

T-1095 was the next agent developed but did not continue into clinical development as it was again nonselective in nature and had safety concerns [57].

By modification in basic structure of phlorizin, other SGLT2-I were developed, including AVE-2268, remogliflozin, sergliflozin, and WAY-123783.

All of them have the glucoside moiety linked to a distal phenolic ring via an O-linkage. Due to susceptibility of O-linkage to degradation by β-glucosidases which reduced their utility, development of more metabolically stable C-linkage SGLT2 inhibitors was prompted with focus on increasing selectivity for SGLT2 versus SGLT1. This led to discovery of dapagliflozin, canagliflozin, empagliflozin, ipragliflozin, BI 44847, and LX 4211 [58, 59].

6. Clinical effects of SGLT2 inhibitors in diabetes mellitus

Currently, there are seven SGLT2 inhibitors approved for clinical use. They are given orally and absorbed by the intestine. Due to higher selectivity for SGLT2 versus SGLT1, inhibition of intestinal SGLT1 can be avoided, though it is still possible at high oral doses. At pharmacological doses, their serum levels achieved are too low to inhibit SGLT1 in other organs (**Table 2**).

Clinical effects observed for different SGLT2-I will be described and discussed together for the sake of clarity.

6.1 Effects on diabetes and metabolism

In T2DM, upregulation of SGLT2 expression increases its T_m by around 20%. SGLT2-I is filtered in glomeruli and inhibits glucose reabsorption in S1 segment of proximal tubule leading to a reduction of 30–50% in T_m of SGLT2 [67].

In the presence of functional SGLT2, less than 10% of glucose is absorbed through SGLT1; therefore, it is expected that SGLT2 inhibitor therapy would lead to around 90% reduction in T_m but the observed decrease of only 30–50% in T_m can be explained by higher amount of SGLT1-mediated glucose reabsorption [70].

Compound	Preparation strength available	SGLT2/SGLT1 selectivity	Reference
Dapagliflozin	5, 10 mg	1200	[60]
Canagliflozin	100, 300 mg	200	[61]
Empagliflozin	10, 25 mg	2500	[62]
Ertugliflozin	5, 15 mg	2000	[63]
Ipragliflozin	25, 50 mg	254	[64]
Luseogliflozin	2.5, 5 mg	1765	[65]
Tofogliflozin	20 mg	2900	[66]

Table 2.
Preparation strength and SGLT2 versus SGLT1 selectivity of various approved SGLT2 inhibitors.

During preclinical studies with animal models of diabetes as well as in clinical studies with both T2DM and T1DM patients, it has been demonstrated that prolonged SGLT2-I therapy decreased fasting and prandial plasma glucose levels, reduced HbA1C, and improved oral glucose tolerance. They also exerted nephroprotective effects, reduced blood pressure, and increased utilization of fatty acid substrates; thus, they also conferred metabolic benefits [68–73].

SGLT2-I have insulin-independent mechanism of action. They can be used both as monotherapy as well as in combination with other OAHs [74, 75]. Clinical trials have shown that SGLT2-I are effective when administered in combination with metformin [74, 76–78], metformin plus sulfonylurea [79], insulin [80], DPP4 inhibitors [77], and thiazolidinediones [75].

SGLT2-I do not increase the risk of hypoglycemia like other OAH agents. The filtered renal glucose load is directly correlated with plasma glucose level, and there is compensatory increase in SGLT1-mediated glucose reabsorption when SGLT2 is blocked [81]. The other mechanism preventing hypoglycemia is the glucagon secretion from pancreatic alpha cells due to SGLT2 inhibition [31].

SGLT2-I therapy in patients with T2DM increases both plasma glucagon and endogenous glucose production. Despite such physiological changes, patients on SGLT2-I have lower plasma glucose levels than those receiving placebo, possibly because of increased glycosuria and improved insulin sensitivity [82, 83].

SGLT2-I administration changes body metabolism and shifts it to enhanced usage of fat for metabolic needs; consequently beta-hydroxybutyrate levels in plasma increase [69]. The metabolic inflexibility characteristically seen in patients with T2DM and nondiabetic insulin-resistant subjects is an inability to switch from predominantly fatty acid oxidation during fasting state to predominantly glucose oxidation in fed state [84]. Lack of variability in measured respiratory quotient (RQ) between fasting and fed states has been observed as an evidence of metabolic inflexibility. SGLT2-I reduce whole body fasting RQ which is indicative of increased oxidation of fatty acids and amino acids, suggesting its partial restoration [85].

As a consequence of improved glucose homoeostasis, SGLT2-I may slow down glucotoxicity-mediated degeneration of beta cells and thus may also slow down the progression of T2DM. Experimental diabetic animal models on SGLT2-I have shown an improvement in both beta cell mass and functions [86]. Improvement in insulin sensitivity is another beneficial aspect [82, 83].

6.2 Effects on blood pressure

Increased urinary excretion of glucose and sodium leads to mild diuresis coupled with urinary sodium loss. Reduction of extracellular volume occurs which has a favorable effect on blood pressure, and the magnitude of the effect is most apparent in patients with preexisting hypertension [87].

Empagliflozin causes a reduction in systolic blood pressure (SBP) of 4–6 mmHg, whereas diastolic blood pressure (DBP) was similar to placebo with no increase in the heart rate [88]. Similarly, canagliflozin at 300 mg/day resulted in a reduction in SBP of 5.1 mmHg [89].

In analysis of 12 studies with dapagliflozin at 10 mg/day, reduction of 4.4 mmHg and 0.5 mmHg in SBP and DBP, respectively, was seen with no increase in the heart rate compared to placebo [90].

6.3 Effects on body weight

On SGLT2-I therapy, initial weight loss could result from osmotic diuresis. However, sustained weight loss over the period is a consequence of renal glucose excretion leading to a caloric deficit of about 280 calories/day. This translates into decrease in body weight by 1–3 kg along with decreased visceral adiposity.

In the EMPA-REG trial, empagliflozin resulted in weight loss of about 2 kg [91]. The average weight loss achieved with dapagliflozin and canagliflozin stands between 1 and 3%, while other studies report a loss more than 5% [92, 93].

6.4 Effects on plasma lipids and plasma uric acid

SGLT2-I therapy has been associated with alteration in serum lipid profile. Small increase in low-density lipoprotein cholesterol (LDL) and high-density lipoprotein cholesterol (HDL) has been observed [76, 78, 94].

Any increase in serum cholesterol is considered to be a risk factor for the development of heart failure and CVDs. However, it may not be relevant clinically, as empagliflozin has been shown to have a protective effect on MACE in EMPA-REG trial [91].

They also promote uric acid excretion and reduce uric acid level in the blood [94] which may contribute to their protective effect on the development of diabetic nephropathy observed in the EMPA-REG renal study [73, 80, 95].

6.5.1 Effects on cardiovascular disease

In EMPA-REG trial, empagliflozin has shown a lower risk for MACE as well as for cardiovascular death and has been found to be protective [88].

In CANVAS Program, canagliflozin has been found to reduce the risk of cardiovascular death or hospitalization for heart failure in patient with a history of T2DM and high CVD risk [96].

Lately, DECLARE-TIMI 58 trial demonstrated the CV safety of dapagliflozin in patients with T2DM who had or were at risk of CVDs. It was found to reduce hospitalization for heart failure as has been seen with other SGLT2-I [97].

Both empagliflozin and canagliflozin has got FDA approval for cardiovascular risk reduction in T2DM patients who are at high risk for such events. The mechanism of cardiovascular protection exerted by SGLT2-I is unknown and seems to be glucose independent. Apart from improved glycemic control, the pleiotropic effects of SGLT2 inhibitors which include their ability to lower blood pressure, reduction in intraglomerular pressure and albuminuria, and amelioration of volume overload are all plausible protective mechanisms.

6.5.2 Effects on liver disease

T2DM affects metabolism in the liver and may manifest as hepatic steatosis and nonalcoholic steatohepatitis (NASH). NASH increases the risk of hepatocellular carcinoma and may result in liver cirrhosis also.

In preclinical studies on rodent models, SGLT2-I have been found to ameliorate nonalcoholic fatty liver disease (NAFLD) and NASH [70–72]. Although SGLT2-I are metabolized by the liver, studies involving patient with mild or moderate hepatic impairment showed dapagliflozin and empagliflozin were well tolerated and required no dose adjustments [98, 99].

Canagliflozin has shown improvement in serum aminotransferases and gamma-glutamyl transferase levels in patients with T2DM [100]. In humans, ipragliflozin has shown reduction in liver fat in patients with T2DM and NAFLD [101]. Empagliflozin addition to the standard treatment of T2DM and NAFLD significantly reduced liver fat, and improved ALT levels were seen [102].

6.5.3 Effects on kidney disease

The kidney is the main target of action for SGLT2-I. Findings from animal models suggest it to be protective against development of diabetic nephropathy which exceeds the nephroprotective effect achieved secondary to improved glycemic control. During early stage of nephropathy, empagliflozin has been shown to prevent glomerular hyperfiltration, attenuate diabetes-associated renal growth, improve expression of inflammation markers, and reduce albuminuria in animal models [24].

Progression of nephropathy was slowed by luseogliflozin in T2DN rats, a genetic model of T2DM associated with severe nephropathy. It also prevents GFR decline and attenuates focal glomerulosclerosis, tubular necrosis, tubulointerstitial fibrosis, and progressive proteinuria [103].

Reduction in estimated GFR and nephroprotective effects has been reported with SGLT2-I in patients with DM [73, 80, 104]. Empagliflozin has been found to attenuate glomerular hyperfiltration in humans. It also reduces micro- and macroalbuminuria, and the effects are independent of the improved glycemic effect [105]. In CANVAS trial, canagliflozin has been found to reduce albuminuria and the albumin-to-creatinine ratio when compared with placebo [106].

Results from a recent meta-analysis have indicated that SGLT2 inhibition preserves renal function in patient with or without renal impairment. They slow down the progression of albuminuria and reduce urinary albumin-to-creatinine ratio in addition to reducing the risk of doubling of the serum creatinine level, initiation of kidney transplant, and death from kidney disease in patient with T2DM with or without history of renal impairment [107].

6.6 Risks for adverse drug effects and restrictions of application

6.6.1 Genital and urinary infections

Increased risk of GMI and urinary tract infections (UTI) are seen in DM due to hyperglycemia and glucosuria. SGLT2-I therapy has been associated with increased risks for GMIs and UTIs. Women otherwise also are more commonly affected than men, and SGLT2-I therapy further increases the risk in them.

When treated with canagliflozin for 4 months, around 10.4% of women and 4.2% of men developed GMIs compared to 3.2% of women and 0.6% of men treated with placebo [108]. Most of the cases were of mild to moderate severity and could be treated with standard antifungal agents successfully.

Canagliflozin therapy in T2DM has been associated with UTIs in 8.7% of women compared to 7.7% treated with placebo. Figures for men were 1.4% versus 0.6%, respectively [109]. Similar findings were reported from pooled analysis of four studies (n = 2477) using empagliflozin. It was concluded that GMI were more common with empagliflozin than placebo (approximately 4 versus 1%, respectively); however, the frequency of UTI was about 8–9% for each [110].

Safety data from meta-analysis of eight studies using canagliflozin and dapagliflozin found that UTIs were more common with SGLT2-I as compared to other OAH (odds ratio, 1.42 [95% CI 1.06, 1.90]) as were GMI (odds ratio, 5.06 [95% CI 3.44, 7.45]) [111].

These studies suggests that most UTIs were mild to moderate, responded well to standard antimicrobial therapy, and rarely led to SGLT2-I discontinuation [112].

6.6.2 Euglycemic ketoacidosis

SGLT2-I therapy has been observed to be associated with small number of cases with EKA during treatment of T1DM and insulin-deficient T2DM [113].

In CANVAS study, the incidence rates were 0.5 per 1000 patient years with canagliflozin 100 mg, 0.8 per 1000 patient years with canagliflozin 300 mg, and 0.2 per 1000 patient years with comparator [114]. In the EMPA-REG trial, the incidence rates were 0.5 and 0.2 per 1000 patient years with empagliflozin 10 and 25 mg, respectively, and 1.2 per 1000 patient years in placebo group [88]. In DECLARE-TIMI 58, using dapagliflozin, the corresponding rates were 0.3%, whereas 0.1% occurred among placebo-treated group [97].

Majority of the cases have been reported from clinical practice rather than trials and have occurred in patients on exogenous insulin. Reduction in insulin dose on starting SGLT2-I has been observed in them. Usually they present with classical diabetic ketoacidosis (DKA) features. However, some cases may present atypically with lower-than-expected hyperglycemia, and it can go unrecognized.

Almost all cases occurred in patients challenged with metabolically stressful events and common precipitants such as surgery, myocardial infarction, stroke, extensive exercise, severe infections, and prolonged fasting.

Low serum bicarbonate and positive urinary ketones may be suggestive but may be inaccurate; therefore, direct measurement of serum betahydroxybutyrate level to confirm the diagnosis of EKA has been recommended by the AACE. Once the diagnosis of EKA is confirmed, SGLT2-I should be discontinued, and DKA protocol should be followed [115].

The increased risk of EKA associated with SGLT2-I therapy may be explained by absolute or relative insulin deficiency, increased glucagon secretion, and stimulation of lipolysis and ketogenesis; however, other ketogenic factors are also involved [31, 69].

Most cases of EKA have occurred in patients with T1DM, which is an off-label use of these agents that is not an FDA-approved indication. Because insulin deficiency may be the most important contributing factor, the AACE recommends against stopping insulin or decreasing the dose excessively. The risk of EKA has recently been shown in the EASE Trial to be dose dependent as lower doses of empagliflozin 2.5 mg were shown to be associated with lower rates of DKA, compared to 10 and 25 mg, respectively [116].

Although not approved for treatment of T1DM and SGLT2-I use is still off-label in T1DM, the AACE encourages clinical trials due to their promising effect on glycemic control in this population [115].

6.6.3 SGLT2 inhibitors and risk of limb amputations

Canagliflozin significantly reduced the risk of CV events by 14% but increased the risk of lower limb amputation in patients with T2DM and high CVD risk (hazard ratio 1.97) versus placebo as seen in CANVAS trial [114].

In the EMAP REG trial using empagliflozin, in T2DM patient with established CVD, the rate of lower limb amputation was similar to placebo group [88].

Recently in DECLARE-TIMI 58 trial, the rate of amputation was similar between the dapagliflozin- and placebo-treated patient (hazard ratio 1.09) [97].

In a recent report, canagliflozin, but not dapagliflozin or empagliflozin, was associated with a higher risk of amputation in a pharmacovigilance analysis using the US FDA Adverse Event Reporting System [117].

Presently the evidence may not be enough to explain a precise causal relationship between canagliflozin and amputation. Neither the underlying mechanisms are currently known, nor do we know whether it is specifically related to canagliflozin. As amputation carries a negative impact on patient's clinical course, understanding predisposing factors and mechanisms of amputation will be crucial to maximize the benefits of SGLT2 inhibitors in clinical practice [117].

6.6.4 *Effect on bone health*

In CANVAS study, patients treated with canagliflozin had about six additional cases of bone fracture compared to those receiving placebo. However, such an effect could not be replicated in other trials of canagliflozin [118].

Canagliflozin is associated with a small but statistically significant decrease in total hip bone mineral density (BMD) but no statistically significant change in BMD at other sites and without any meaningful changes in most biomarkers of bone turnover [118].

No significant changes in bone density or increase in rate of fracture were observed with dapagliflozin in patients with DM and normal or mildly impaired renal function, but more fractures were observed in dapagliflozin-treated patients with moderate renal impairment (eGFR $\leq$30–60 mL/min/1.73 m^2) [104]. Empagliflozin however did not show any clear evidence of increase fracture rates in people with T2DM [119].

Furthermore, the absence of SGLT2 in bone or bone marrow makes direct cause-effect hypothesis unlikely. It is known that SGLT2-I induce osmotic diuresis leading to volume depletion which may increase the susceptibility to falls. An increase in fall-related fractures cannot be ruled out as a possible explanation. The exact reason and mechanism are unknown at this time and may possibly be related to factors extrinsic to bone health [28].

Pending further evidence, the US FDA has revised the label of canagliflozin with new warning in September 2015.

6.4.5 *Restrictions of application*

SGLT2-I are prescribed as once daily oral pill due to their long elimination half-life. They are metabolized in the liver, and inactive metabolites are formed mainly due to glucuronidation.

They are also eliminated partially by renal excretion of parent drugs. Thus, dose adjustment is needed in patients with hepatic and/or renal disorders. They are contraindicated in severe chronic kidney disease.

7. Conclusion

SGLT2-I are a unique emerging class of OAH agents that has addressed fundamental aspects of the unmet needs that challenge physicians treating T2DM patients, such as increased risk of hypoglycemia and weight gain that are usually noticed with other agents such as insulin. On the contrary, SGLT2-I therapy in T2DM is associated with very low risk of hypoglycemia and also promotes weight loss. Moreover, SGLT2-I have been shown to reduce the risk of MACE, all-cause mortality, and hospitalization for heart failure. They have additional renal protective properties besides reducing SBP. In fact, their mode of action through prevention of glucose reabsorption in the kidney makes them work independently from the pancreas, bypassing the problem of progressive beta cell failure that happens in most patients with T2DM over time, and this gives them longer durability. They can be used regardless of duration of disease and can be used as monotherapy as well as in combination as they have been shown to complement actions of other OAH agents including insulin. Considering their unique mechanism of action, they may be useful in impaired glucose tolerance and prediabetes also. The major side effects drawbacks of SGLT2-I is the increased rate of GMI. Another important side effect of SGLT2-I is EKA in T2DM patients during stress and following surgery as well as in T1DM, which is an off-label use of these medications and seems to be dose dependent. Future drug developments should focus on finding the least effective dose with the least side effects.

Conflict of interest

Authors declare that there is no conflict of interest. No fund or grant was received in any form for this work.

Author details

Maswood M. Ahmad*, Imad Addin Brema and Mussa H. Almalki
Obesity Endocrine and Metabolism Center, King Fahad Medical City, Riyadh, Saudi Arabia

*Address all correspondence to: saadmaswood@gmail.com

References

[1] Unger RH, Cherrington AD. Glucagonocentric restructuring of diabetes: A pathophysiologic and therapeutic makeover. The Journal of Clinical Investigation. 2012;**122**(1):4-12

[2] Cho NH, Shaw JE, Karuranga S, Huang Y, da Rocha Fernandes JD, Ohlrogge AW, et al. IDF diabetes atlas: Global estimates of diabetes prevalence for 2017 and projections for 2045. Diabetes Research and Clinical Practice. 2018;**138**:271-281

[3] American Diabetes Association (ADA). Standard of medical care in diabetes—2018. Diabetes Care. 2018;**41**(Supplement 1):S1-S159. https://doi.org/10.2337/dc18-Sint01

[4] Davies MJ, D'Alessio DA, Fradkin J, Kernan WN, Mathieu C, Mingrone G, et al. Management of hyperglycaemia in type 2 diabetes, 2018. A consensus report by the American Diabetes Association (ADA) and the European Association for the Study of Diabetes (EASD). Diabetologia. 2018;**61**(12):2461-2498

[5] Centers for Disease Control and Prevention. National diabetes statistics report: Estimates of diabetes and its burden in the United States, 2014. Atlanta, GA: US Department of Health and Human Services; 2014. Available from: https://www.cdc.gov/diabetes/pdfs/data/2014-report-estimates-of-diabetes-and-its-burden-in-the-united-states.pdf [Accessed: November 20, 2018]

[6] Stratton IM, Adler AI, Neil HA, Matthews DR, Manley SE, Cull CA, et al. Association of glycaemia with macrovascular and microvascular complications of type 2 diabetes (UKPDS 35): Prospective observational study. British Medical Journal. 2000;**321**(7258):405-412

[7] UK Prospective Diabetes Study (UKPDS) Group. Intensive blood-glucose control with sulphonylureas or insulin compared with conventional treatment and risk of complications in patients with type 2 diabetes (UKPDS 33). The Lancet. 1998;**352**(9131):837-853

[8] ADVANCE Collaborative Group. Intensive blood glucose control and vascular outcomes in patients with type 2 diabetes. New England Journal of Medicine. 2008;**358**(24):2560-2572

[9] Action to Control Cardiovascular Risk in Diabetes Study Group. Effects of intensive glucose lowering in type 2 diabetes. New England Journal of Medicine. 2008;**358**(24):2545-2559

[10] Holman RR, Paul SK, Bethel MA, Matthews DR, Neil HA. 10-year follow-up of intensive glucose control in type 2 diabetes. New England Journal of Medicine. 2008;**359**(15):1577-1589

[11] Duckworth W, Abraira C, Moritz T, Reda D, Emanuele N, Reaven PD, et al. Glucose control and vascular complications in veterans with type 2 diabetes. New England Journal of Medicine. 2009;**360**(2):129-139

[12] DeFronzo RA. From the triumvirate to the "ominous octet": A new paradigm for the treatment of type 2 diabetes mellitus. Clinical Diabetology. 2009;**10**(3):101-128

[13] Ali MK, Bullard KM, Saaddine JB, Cowie CC, Imperatore G, Gregg EW. Achievement of goals in US diabetes care, 1999-2010. New England Journal of Medicine. 2013;**368**(17):1613-1624

[14] Singh S, Loke YK, Furberg CD. Long-term risk of cardiovascular events with rosiglitazone: A meta-analysis. Journal of the American Medical Association. 2007;**298**(10):1189-1195

[15] US FDA. Guidance for Industry Diabetes Mellitus—Evaluating Cardiovascular Risk in New Antidiabetic Therapies to Treat Type 2 Diabetes. 2008. Available from: www.fda.gov/downloads/drugs/guidancecomplianceregulatory information/guidances/ucm071627.pdf [Accessed 4 July 2010] 2016. Last accessed 21 November 2018

[16] Marks J, Carvou NJ, Debnam ES, Srai SK, Unwin RJ. Diabetes increases facilitative glucose uptake and GLUT2 expression at the rat proximal tubule brush border membrane. The Journal of Physiology. 2003;**553**(1):137-145

[17] Gorboulev V, Schürmann A, Vallon V, Kipp H, Jaschke A, Klessen D, et al. Na^+-D-glucose cotransporter SGLT1 is pivotal for intestinal glucose absorption and glucose-dependent incretin secretion. Diabetes. 2012;**61**(1):187-196

[18] Cho YM, Fujita Y, Kieffer TJ. Glucagon-like peptide-1: Glucose homeostasis and beyond. Annual Review of Physiology. 2014;**76**:535-559

[19] Wood IS, Trayhurn P. Glucose transporters (GLUT and SGLT): Expanded families of sugar transport proteins. British Journal of Nutrition. 2003;**89**(1):3-9

[20] .Wright EM, Hirayama BA, Loo DF. Active sugar transport in health and disease. Journal of Internal Medicine. 2007;**261**(1):32-43s

[21] Turk E, Martín MG, Wright EM. Structure of the human Na^+/glucose cotransporter gene SGLT1. Journal of Biological Chemistry. 1994;**269**(21):15204-15209

[22] Thomson SC, Deng A, Bao D, Satriano J, Blantz RC, Vallon V. Ornithine decarboxylase, kidney size, and the tubular hypothesis of glomerular hyperfiltration in experimental diabetes. The Journal of Clinical Investigation. 2001;**107**(2):217-224

[23] Vallon V, Rose M, Gerasimova M, Satriano J, Platt KA, Koepsell H, et al. Knockout of Na-glucose transporter SGLT2 attenuates hyperglycemia and glomerular hyperfiltration but not kidney growth or injury in diabetes mellitus. American Journal of Physiology-Renal Physiology. 2012;**304**(2):F156-F167

[24] Vallon V, Gerasimova M, Rose MA, Masuda T, Satriano J, Mayoux E, et al. SGLT2 inhibitor empagliflozin reduces renal growth and albuminuria in proportion to hyperglycemia and prevents glomerular hyperfiltration in diabetic Akita mice. American Journal of Physiology—Renal Physiology. 2013;**306**(2):F194-F204

[25] Turk E, Zabel B, Mundlos S, Dyer J, Wright EM. Glucose/galactose malabsorption caused by a defect in the Na^+/glucose cotransporter. Nature. 1991;**350**(6316):354

[26] Santer R, Calado J. Familial renal glucosuria and SGLT2: From a mendelian trait to a therapeutic target. Clinical Journal of the American Society of Nephrology. 2010;**5**(1):133-141

[27] Santer R, Kinner M, Lassen CL, Schneppenheim R, Eggert P, Bald M, et al. Molecular analysis of the SGLT2 gene in patients with renal glucosuria. Journal of the American Society of Nephrology. 2003;**14**(11):2873-2882

[28] Wright EM, Loo DD, Hirayama BA. Biology of human sodium glucose transporters. Physiological Reviews. 2011;**91**(2):733-794

[29] Vrhovac I, Eror DB, Klessen D, Burger C, Breljak D, Kraus O, et al. Localizations of Na^+-D-glucose cotransporters SGLT1 and SGLT2 in human kidney and of SGLT1 in human small intestine, liver, lung, and heart.

Pflügers Archiv-European Journal of Physiology. 2015;**467**(9):1881-1898

[30] Chen J, Williams S, Ho S, Loraine H, Hagan D, Whaley JM, et al. Quantitative PCR tissue expression profiling of the human SGLT2 gene and related family members. Diabetes Therapy. 2010;**1**(2):57-92

[31] Bonner C, Kerr-Conte J, Gmyr V, Queniat G, Moerman E, Thévenet J, et al. Inhibition of the glucose transporter SGLT2 with dapagliflozin in pancreatic alpha cells triggers glucagon secretion. Nature Medicine. 2015;**21**(5):512

[32] Zhou L, Cryan EV, D'Andrea MR, Belkowski S, Conway BR, Demarest KT. Human cardiomyocytes express high level of Na+/glucose cotransporter 1 (SGLT1). Journal of Cellular Biochemistry. 2003;**90**(2):339-346

[33] Poppe R, Karbach U, Gambaryan S, Wiesinger H, Lutzenburg M, Kraemer M, et al. Expression of the Na^+-D-glucose cotransporter SGLT1 in neurons. Journal of Neurochemistry. 1997;**69**(1):84-94

[34] Hirayama BA, Lostao MP, Panayotova-Heiermann MA, Loo DD, Turk ER, Wright EM. Kinetic and specificity differences between rat, human, and rabbit Na^+-glucose cotransporters (SGLT-1). American Journal of Physiology-Gastrointestinal and Liver Physiology. 1996;**270**(6): G919-G926

[35] Linda CH, Turner JR, Buret AG. LPS/CD14 activation triggers SGLT-1-mediated glucose uptake and cell rescue in intestinal epithelial cells via early apoptotic signals upstream of caspase-3. Experimental Cell Research. 2006;**312**(17):3276-3286

[36] Ikari A, Nagatani Y, Tsukimoto M, Harada H, Miwa M, Takagi K. Sodium-dependent glucose transporter reduces peroxynitrite and cell injury caused by cisplatin in renal tubular epithelial cells. Biochimica et Biophysica Acta (BBA)—Biomembranes. 2005;**1717**(2):109-117

[37] O'Malley D, Reimann F, Simpson AK, Gribble FM. Sodium-coupled glucose cotransporters contribute to hypothalamic glucose sensing. Diabetes. 2006;**55**(12):3381-3386

[38] Yamazaki Y, Ogihara S, Harada S, Tokuyama S. Activation of cerebral sodium-glucose transporter type 1 function mediated by post-ischemic hyperglycemia exacerbates the development of cerebral ischemia. Neuroscience. 2015;**310**:674-685

[39] Harada S, Fujita W, Shichi K, Tokuyama S. The development of glucose intolerance after focal cerebral ischemia participates in subsequent neuronal damage. Brain Research. 2009;**1279**:174-181

[40] Kashiwagi Y, Nagoshi T, Yoshino T, Tanaka TD, Ito K, Harada T, et al. Expression of SGLT1 in human hearts and impairment of cardiac glucose uptake by phlorizin during ischemia-reperfusion injury in mice. PLoS One. 2015;**10**(6):e0130605

[41] Balteau M, Tajeddine N, de Meester C, Ginion A, Des Rosiers C, Brady NR, et al. NADPH oxidase activation by hyperglycaemia in cardiomyocytes is independent of glucose metabolism but requires SGLT1. Cardiovascular Research. 2011;**92**(2):237-246

[42] Basset G, Crone C, Saumon G. Fluid absorption by rat lung in situ: Pathways for sodium entry in the luminal membrane of alveolar epithelium. The Journal of Physiology. 1987;**384**:325-345

[43] Bhavsar SK, Singh Y, Sharma P, Khairnar V, Hosseinzadeh Z, Zhang S, et al. Expression of JAK3 sensitive Na^+ coupled glucose carrier SGLT1 in activated cytotoxic T lymphocytes.

Cellular Physiology and Biochemistry. 2016;**39**(3):1209-1228

[44] Rhoads DB, Rosenbaum DH, Unsal H, Isselbacher KJ, Levitsky LL. Circadian periodicity of intestinal Na^+/glucose cotransporter 1 mRNA levels is transcriptionally regulated. Journal of Biological Chemistry. 1998;**273**(16):9510-9516

[45] Barfull A, Garriga C, Tauler A, Planas JM. Regulation of SGLT1 expression in response to Na^+ intake. American Journal of Physiology-Regulatory, Integrative and Comparative Physiology. 2002;**282**(3):R738-R743

[46] Dyer J, Wood IS, Palejwala A, Ellis A, Shirazi-Beechey SP. Expression of monosaccharide transporters in intestine of diabetic humans. American Journal of Physiology—Gastrointestinal and Liver Physiology. 2002;**282**(2):G241-G248

[47] Kekuda R, Saha P, Sundaram U. Role of Sp1 and HNF1 transcription factors in SGLT1 regulation during chronic intestinal inflammation. American Journal of Physiology—Gastrointestinal and Liver Physiology. 2008;**294**(6):G1354-G1361

[48] Sabolić I, Vrhovac I, Eror DB, Gerasimova M, Rose M, Breljak D, et al. Expression of Na^+-D-glucose cotransporter SGLT2 in rodents is kidney-specific and exhibits sex and species differences. American Journal of Physiology—Cell Physiology. 2012;**302**(8):C1174-C1188

[49] Vallon V. The proximal tubule in the pathophysiology of the diabetic kidney. American Journal of Physiology—Regulatory, Integrative and Comparative Physiology. 2010;**300**(5):R1009-R1022

[50] Ruggenenti P, Porrini EL, Gaspari F, Motterlini N, Cannata A, Carrara F, et al. Glomerular hyperfiltration and renal disease progression in type 2 diabetes. Diabetes Care. 2012:DC_112189

[51] Zhang Q, Ramracheya R, Lahmann C, Tarasov A, Bengtsson M, Braha O, et al. Role of K ATP channels in glucose-regulated glucagon secretion and impaired counterregulation in type 2 diabetes. Cell Metabolism. 2013;**18**(6):871-882

[52] Zhao Y, Gao P, Sun F, Li Q, Chen J, Yu H, et al. Sodium intake regulates glucose homeostasis through the PPARδ/adiponectin-mediated SGLT2 pathway. Cell Metabolism. 2016;**23**(4):699-711

[53] Han HJ, Lee YJ, Park SH, Lee JH, Taub M. High glucose-induced oxidative stress inhibits Na^+/glucose cotransporter activity in renal proximal tubule cells. American Journal of Physiology—Renal Physiology. 2005;**288**(5):F988-F996

[54] Rafiq K, Fujisawa Y, Sherajee SJ, Rahman A, Sufiun A, Kobori H, et al. Role of the renal sympathetic nerve in renal glucose metabolism during the development of type 2 diabetes in rats. Diabetologia. 2015;**58**(12):2885-2898

[55] Coady MJ, El Tarazi A, Santer R, Bissonnette P, Sasseville LJ, Calado J, et al. MAP17 is a necessary activator of renal Na+/glucose cotransporter SGLT2. Journal of the American Society of Nephrology. 2017;**28**(1):85-93

[56] Rossetti L, Shulman GI, Zawalich W, DeFronzo RA. Effect of chronic hyperglycemia on in vivo insulin secretion in partially pancreatectomized rats. The Journal of Clinical Investigation. 1987;**80**(4):1037-1044

[57] Oku A, Ueta K, Arakawa K, Ishihara T, Nawano M, Kuronuma Y, et al. T-1095, an inhibitor of renal Na^+-glucose cotransporters, may provide a novel approach to treating diabetes. Diabetes. 1999;**48**(9):1794-1800

[58] Katsuno K, Fujimori Y, Takemura Y, Hiratochi M, Itoh F, Komatsu Y, et al. Sergliflozin, a novel selective inhibitor of low-affinity sodium glucose cotransporter (SGLT2), validates the critical role of SGLT2 in renal glucose reabsorption and modulates plasma glucose level. Journal of Pharmacology and Experimental Therapeutics. 2007;**320**(1):323-330

[59] Dobbins RL, O'Connor-Semmes R, Kapur A, Kapitza C, Golor G, Mikoshiba I, et al. Remogliflozin etabonate, a selective inhibitor of the sodium-dependent transporter 2 reduces serum glucose in type 2 diabetes mellitus patients. Diabetes, Obesity and Metabolism. 2012;**14**(1):15-22

[60] Han S, Hagan DL, Taylor JR, Xin L, Meng W, Biller SA, et al. Dapagliflozin, a selective SGLT2 inhibitor, improves glucose homeostasis in normal and diabetic rats. Diabetes. 2008

[61] Ohgaki R, Wei L, Yamada K, Hara T, Kuriyama C, Okuda S, et al. Interaction of the sodium/glucose cotransporter (SGLT) 2 inhibitor canagliflozin with SGLT1 and SGLT2: Inhibition kinetics, sidedness of action, and transporter-associated incorporation accounting for its pharmacodynamic and pharmacokinetic features. Journal of Pharmacology and Experimental Therapeutics. 2016;**358**(1):94-102

[62] Grempler R, Thomas L, Eckhardt M, Himmelsbach F, Sauer A, Sharp DE, et al. Empagliflozin, a novel selective sodium glucose cotransporter-2 (SGLT-2) inhibitor: Characterisation and comparison with other SGLT-2 inhibitors. Diabetes, Obesity and Metabolism. 2012;**14**(1):83-90

[63] Cinti F, Moffa S, Impronta F, Cefalo CM, Sun VA, Sorice GP, et al. Spotlight on ertugliflozin and its potential in the treatment of type 2 diabetes: Evidence to date. Drug Design, Development and Therapy. 2017;**11**:2905

[64] Tahara A, Kurosaki E, Yokono M, Yamajuku D, Kihara R, Hayashizaki Y, et al. Pharmacological profile of ipragliflozin (ASP1941), a novel selective SGLT2 inhibitor, in vitro and in vivo. Naunyn-Schmiedeberg's Archives of Pharmacology. 2012;**385**(4):423-436

[65] Yamamoto K, Uchida S, Kitano K, Fukuhara N, Okumura-Kitajima L, Gunji E, et al. TS-071 is a novel, potent and selective renal sodium-glucose cotransporter 2 (SGLT2) inhibitor with anti-hyperglycaemic activity. British Journal of Pharmacology. 2011;**164**(1):181-191

[66] Suzuki M, Honda K, Fukazawa M, Ozawa K, Hagita H, Kawai T, et al. Tofogliflozin, a potent and highly specific sodium/glucose cotransporter 2 inhibitor, improves glycemic control in diabetic rats and mice. Journal of Pharmacology and Experimental Therapeutics. 2012;**341**(3):692-701

[67] DeFronzo RA, Hompesch M, Kasichayanula S, Liu X, Hong Y, Pfister M, et al. Characterization of renal glucose reabsorption in response to dapagliflozin in healthy subjects and subjects with type 2 diabetes. Diabetes Care. 2013:DC_130387

[68] Gallo LA, Wright EM, Vallon V. Probing SGLT2 as a therapeutic target for diabetes: Basic physiology and consequences. Diabetes and Vascular Disease Research. 2015;**12**(2):78-89

[69] Ferrannini E, Baldi S, Frascerra S, Astiarraga B, Heise T, Bizzotto R, et al. Shift to fatty substrates utilization in response to sodium-glucose co-transporter-2 inhibition in nondiabetic subjects and type 2 diabetic patients. Diabetes. 2016:db151356

[70] Komiya C, Tsuchiya K, Shiba K, Miyachi Y, Furuke S, Shimazu N, et al. Ipragliflozin improves hepatic steatosis in obese mice and liver dysfunction in

type 2 diabetic patients irrespective of body weight reduction. PLoS One. 2016 Mar 15;**11**(3):e0151511

[71] Qiang S, Nakatsu Y, Seno Y, Fujishiro M, Sakoda H, Kushiyama A, et al. Treatment with the SGLT2 inhibitor luseogliflozin improves nonalcoholic steatohepatitis in a rodent model with diabetes mellitus. Diabetology & Metabolic Syndrome. 2015;**7**(1):104

[72] Tahara A, Kurosaki E, Yokono M, Yamajuku D, Kihara R, Hayashizaki Y, et al. Effects of SGLT2 selective inhibitor ipragliflozin on hyperglycemia, hyperlipidemia, hepatic steatosis, oxidative stress, inflammation, and obesity in type 2 diabetic mice. European Journal of Pharmacology. 2013;**715**(1-3):246-255

[73] Wanner C, Inzucchi SE, Lachin JM, Fitchett D, von Eynatten M, Mattheus M, et al. Empagliflozin and progression of kidney disease in type 2 diabetes. New England Journal of Medicine. 2016;**375**(4):323-334

[74] Rosenstock J, Chuck L, González-Ortiz M, Merton K, Craig J, Capuano G, et al. Initial combination therapy with canagliflozin plus metformin versus each component as monotherapy for drug-naive type 2 diabetes. Diabetes Care. 2016:dc151736

[75] DeFronzo RA, Chilton R, Norton L, Clarke G, Ryder RE, Abdul-Ghani M. Revitalization of pioglitazone: The optimum agent to be combined with a sodium-glucose co-transporter-2 inhibitor. Diabetes, Obesity and Metabolism. 2016;**18**(5):454-462

[76] Nauck MA, Del Prato S, Meier JJ, Durán-García S, Rohwedder K, Elze M, et al. Dapagliflozin versus glipizide as add-on therapy in patients with type 2 diabetes who have inadequate glycemic control with metformin: A randomized, 52-week, double-blind, active-controlled noninferiority trial. Diabetes Care. 2011:DC_110606

[77] DeFronzo RA, Lewin A, Patel S, Liu D, Kaste R, Woerle HJ, et al. Combination of empagliflozin and linagliptin as second-line therapy in subjects with type 2 diabetes inadequately controlled on metformin. Diabetes Care. 2015:dc142364

[78] Leiter LA, Yoon KH, Arias P, Langslet G, Xie J, Balis DA, et al. Canagliflozin provides durable glycemic improvements and body weight reduction over 104 weeks versus glimepiride in patients with type 2 diabetes on metformin: A randomized, double-blind, phase 3 study. Diabetes Care. 2015;**38**(3):355-364

[79] Schernthaner G, Gross JL, Rosenstock J, Guarisco M, Fu M, Yee J, et al. Canagliflozin compared with sitagliptin for patients with type 2 diabetes who do not have adequate glycemic control with metformin plus sulfonylurea: A 52-week randomized trial. Diabetes Care. 2013:DC_122491

[80] Wilding JP, Woo V, Soler NG, Pahor A, Sugg J, Rohwedder K, et al. Long-term efficacy of dapagliflozin in patients with type 2 diabetes mellitus receiving high doses of insulin: A randomized trial. Annals of Internal Medicine. 2012;**156**(6):405-415

[81] Vallon V. The mechanisms and therapeutic potential of SGLT2 inhibitors in diabetes mellitus. Annual Review of Medicine. 2015;**66**:255-270

[82] Ferrannini E, Muscelli E, Frascerra S, Baldi S, Mari A, Heise T, et al. Metabolic response to sodium-glucose cotransporter 2 inhibition in type 2 diabetic patients. The Journal of Clinical Investigation. 2014;**124**(2):499-508

[83] Merovci A, Solis-Herrera C, Daniele G, Eldor R, Fiorentino TV, Tripathy D, et al. Dapagliflozin

improves muscle insulin sensitivity but enhances endogenous glucose production. The Journal of Clinical Investigation. 2014;**124**(2):509-514

[84] Storlien L, Oakes ND, Kelley DE. Metabolic flexibility. Proceedings of the Nutrition Society. 2004;**63**(2):363-368

[85] Daniele G, Xiong J, Solis-Herrera C, Merovci A, Eldor R, Tripathy D, et al. Dapagliflozin enhances fat oxidation and ketone production in patients with type 2 diabetes. Diabetes Care. 2016:dc152688

[86] Cheng ST, Chen L, Li SY, Mayoux E, Leung PS. The effects of empagliflozin, an SGLT2 inhibitor, on pancreatic β-cell mass and glucose homeostasis in type 1 diabetes. PLoS One. 2016;**11**(1):e0147391

[87] Heerspink HJ, Perkins BA, Fitchett DH, Husain M, Cherney DZ. Sodium glucose cotransporter 2 inhibitors in the treatment of diabetes: Cardiovascular and kidney effects, potential mechanisms and clinical applications. Circulation. 2016. DOI: 10.1161/CIRCULATIONAHA.116.021887

[88] Zinman B, Wanner C, Lachin JM, Fitchett D, Bluhmki E, Hantel S, et al. Empagliflozin, cardiovascular outcomes, and mortality in type 2 diabetes. New England Journal of Medicine. 2015;**373**(22):2117-2128

[89] Baker WL, Smyth LR, Riche DM, Bourret EM, Chamberlin KW, White WB. Effects of sodium-glucose co-transporter 2 inhibitors on blood pressure: A systematic review and meta-analysis. Journal of the American Society of Hypertension. 2014;**8**(4):262-275

[90] Sjostrom CD, Sugg J, Tjoen C, Salsali A, Ptaszynska A, Parikh S. Pilot analysis of the effect of the SGLT2 inhibitor dapagliflozin on blood pressure in patients with type 2 diabetes mellitus: A pooled analysis of placebo controlled trials. European Heart Journal. 2012;**33**:680

[91] Zinman B, Inzucchi SE, Lachin JM, Wanner C, Ferrari R, Fitchett D, et al. Rationale, design, and baseline characteristics of a randomized, placebo-controlled cardiovascular outcome trial of empagliflozin (EMPA-REG OUTCOME™). Cardiovascular Diabetology. 2014;**13**(1):102

[92] Sanz-Serra P, Pedro-Botet J, Flores-Le JR, Benaiges D, Chillarón JJ. Dapagliflozin: Beyond glycemic control in the treatment of type 2 diabetes mellitus. Clinica e Investigacion en Arteriosclerosis: Publicacion Oficial de la Sociedad Espanola de Arteriosclerosis. 2015;**27**(4):205-211

[93] Bode B, Stenlöf K, Harris S, Sullivan D, Fung A, Usiskin K, et al. Long-term efficacy and safety of canagliflozin over 104 weeks in patients aged 55-80 years with type 2 diabetes. Diabetes, Obesity and Metabolism. 2015 Mar;**17**(3):294-303

[94] Kovacs CS, Seshiah V, Swallow R, Jones R, Rattunde H, Woerle HJ, et al. EMPA-REG PIO™ trial investigators. Empagliflozin improves glycaemic and weight control as add-on therapy to pioglitazone or pioglitazone plus metformin in patients with type 2 diabetes: A 24-week, randomized, placebo-controlled trial. Diabetes, Obesity and Metabolism. 2014;**16**(2):147-158

[95] Davies MJ, Trujillo A, Vijapurkar U, Damaraju CV, Meininger G. Effect of canagliflozin on serum uric acid in patients with type 2 diabetes mellitus. Diabetes, Obesity and Metabolism. 2015;**17**(4):426-429

[96] Rådholm K, Figtree G, Perkovic V, Solomon SD, Mahaffey KW, de Zeeuw D,

et al. Canagliflozin and heart failure in type 2 diabetes mellitus: Results from the CANVAS program (Canagliflozin Cardiovascular Assessment Study). Circulation. 2018. DOI: 10.1161/CIRCULATIONAHA.118.034222

[97] Wiviott SD, Raz I, Bonaca MP, Mosenzon O, Kato ET, Cahn A, et al. Dapagliflozin and cardiovascular outcomes in type 2 diabetes. New England Journal of Medicine. 2018

[98] Kasichayanula S, Liu X, Zhang W, Pfister M, LaCreta FP, Boulton DW. Influence of hepatic impairment on the pharmacokinetics and safety profile of dapagliflozin: An open-label, parallel-group, single-dose study. Clinical Therapeutics. 2011;**33**(11):1798-1808

[99] Heise T, Seewaldt-Becker E, Macha S, Hantel S, Pinnetti S, Seman L, et al. Safety, tolerability, pharmacokinetics and pharmacodynamics following 4 weeks' treatment with empagliflozin once daily in patients

[100] Seko Y, Sumida Y, Sasaki K, Itoh Y, Iijima H, Hashimoto T, et al. Effects of canagliflozin, an SGLT2 inhibitor, on hepatic function in Japanese patients with type 2 diabetes mellitus: Pooled and subgroup analyses of clinical trials. Journal of Gastroenterology. 2018;**53**(1):140-151

[101] Takase T, Nakamura A, Miyoshi H, Yamamoto C, Atsumi T. Amelioration of fatty liver index in patients with type 2 diabetes on ipragliflozin: An association with glucose-lowering effects. Endocrine Journal. 2017;**64**(3):363-367

[102] Kuchay MS, Krishan S, Mishra SK, Farooqui KJ, Singh MK, Wasir JS, et al. Effect of empagliflozin on liver fat in patients with type 2 diabetes and nonalcoholic fatty liver disease: A randomized controlled trial (E-LIFT trial). Diabetes Care. 2018:dc180165

[103] Kojima N, Williams JM, Takahashi T, Miyata N, Roman RJ. Effects of a new SGLT2 inhibitor, luseogliflozin, on diabetic nephropathy in T2DN rats. Journal of Pharmacology and Experimental Therapeutics. 2013;**345**(3):464-472

[104] Kohan DE, Fioretto P, Tang W, List JF. Long-term study of patients with type 2 diabetes and moderate renal impairment shows that dapagliflozin reduces weight and blood pressure but does not improve glycemic control. Kidney International. 2014;**85**(4):962-971

[105] Chemey DZ, Perkins BA, Soleymanlou N, Malone M, Lai V, Lee A, et al. Renal hemody-namic effect of sodium-glucose cotransporter 2 inhibition in patients with type I diabetes mellitus. Circulation. 2014;**129**(5):587-597

[106] Neal B, Perkovic V, de Zeeuw D, Mahaffey KW, Fulcher G, Ways K, et al. Efficacy and safety of canagliflozin, an inhibitor of sodium-glucose cotransporter 2, when used in conjunction with insulin therapy in patients with type 2 diabetes. Diabetes Care. 2015;**38**(3):403-411

[107] Seidu S, Kunutsor SK, Cos X, Gillani S, Khunti K. SGLT2 inhibitors and renal outcomes in type 2 diabetes with or without renal impairment: A systematic review and meta-analysis. Primary Care Diabetes. 2018;**12**(3):265-283

[108] Nyirjesy P, Sobel JD, Fung A, Mayer C, Capuano G, Ways K, et al. Genital mycotic infections with canagliflozin, a sodium glucose co-transporter 2 inhibitor, in patients with type 2 diabetes mellitus: A pooled analysis of clinical studies. Current Medical Research and Opinion. 2014;**30**(6):1109-1119

[109] Usiskin K, Kline I, Fung A, Mayer C, Meininger G. Safety

and tolerability of canagliflozin in patients with type 2 diabetes mellitus: Pooled analysis of phase 3 study results. Postgraduate Medicine. 2014;**126**(3):16-34

[110] Kim G, Gerich J, Salsali A, Hach T, Hantel S, Woerle HJ, et al. Empagliflozin (EMPA) increases genital infections but not urinary tract infections (UTIs) in pooled data from four pivotal phase III trials. Diabetologie und Stoffwechsel. 2014;**9**(S 01):P140

[111] Vasilakou D, Karagiannis T, Athanasiadou E, Mainou M, Liakos A, Bekiari E, et al. Sodium-glucose cotransporter 2 inhibitors for type 2 diabetes: A systematic review and meta-analysis. Annals of Internal Medicine. 2013;**159**(4):262-274

[112] Johnsson KM, Ptaszynska A, Schmitz B, Sugg J, Parikh SJ, List JF. Urinary tract infections in patients with diabetes treated with dapagliflozin. Journal of Diabetes and its Complications. 2013;**27**(5):473-478

[113] Ogawa W, Sakaguchi K. Euglycemic diabetic ketoacidosis induced by SGLT2 inhibitors: Possible mechanism and contributing factors. Journal of Diabetes Investigation. 2016;**7**(2):135-138

[114] Erondu N, Desai M, Ways K, Meininger G. Diabetic ketoacidosis and related events in the canagliflozin type 2 diabetes clinical program. Diabetes Care. 2015:dc151251

[115] Handelsman Y, Henry RR, Bloomgarden ZT, Dagogo-Jack S, DeFronzo RA, Einhorn D, et al. American Association of Clinical Endocrinologists and American College of Endocrinology position statement on the association of SGLT-2 inhibitors and diabetic ketoacidosis.

[116] Rosenstock J, Marquard J, Laffel LM, Neubacher D, Kaspers S, Cherney DZ, et al. Empagliflozin as adjunctive to insulin therapy in type 1 diabetes: The EASE trials. Diabetes Care. 2018;**41**(12):2560-2569

[117] Fadini GP, Avogaro A. SGLT2 inhibitors and amputations in the US FDA adverse event reporting system. The Lancet Diabetes & Endocrinology. 2017;**5**(9):680-681

[118] Bilezikian JP, Watts NB, Usiskin K, Polidori D, Fung A, Sullivan D, et al. Evaluation of bone mineral density and bone biomarkers in patients with type 2 diabetes treated with canagliflozin. The Journal of Clinical Endocrinology. 2016;**101**(1):44-51

[119] Wanner C, Toto RD, Gerich J, Hach T, Salsali A, Kim G. No increase in bone fractures with empagliflozin (EMPA) in a pooled analysis of more than 11,000 patients with type 2 diabetes (T2DM). Journal of the American Society of Nephrology. 2013;**24**(Suppl):S205A

Chapter 6

Newer Modalities in the Treatment of Type 2 Diabetes Mellitus: Focus on Technology

Alan B. Schorr

Abstract

This chapter will focus on the technological advances for individuals with Type 2 diabetes mellitus and their effect on treatment, control of blood glucoses and possible improvement in lifestyle and decreasing complications. This is a general overview of technological improvements and not an outline for specific patient care. Various technologies will be discussed and the outlook for future improvements outlined.

Keywords: CSII-continuous subcutaneous insulin infusion, CGM-continuous glucose monitoring, HbA1C, MDI-multiple dose injection, smart pen

1. Introduction

During the past 30 years, there has been significant advances in technology for the treatment of patients with Diabetes Mellitus. Most of these advances have focused on patients with Type 1 diabetes mellitus. The perception has been that individuals with Type 2 diabetes mellitus have not needed these advances or that they are not appropriate for a population that does not always require insulin.

Type 2 diabetes mellitus is a disease which is multifactorial: linked to metabolic derangements, Obesity, dietary behavior along with lifestyle issues particularly those individuals who are Sedentary [1, 2]. Given these factors, technology has been considered as adjunct therapeutic modalities to use in addition modification of diet, education, medications and lifestyle changes.

2. Insulin pump therapy (CSII)

Continuous Subcutaneous Insulin Infusion (CSII) has been utilized since the 1970s for the treatment of Diabetes Mellitus. The first insulin pumps were extremely large and bulky. Dr. Arnold Kadish devised a backpack insulin pump in the 1960s, but it proved to be less than optimal for everyday use. Dean Kamen in the late 1970s developed a more practical portable insulin pump which was eventually produced by Baxter called the Auto Syringe. This was the initial insulin pump that this author utilized in the early 1908s. Insulin pumps have evolved significantly over the past 40 years becoming smaller, more precise in the delivery of insulin doses and more reliable than their older versions [3]. During the 1980s to early 2000s, there were several companies providing insulin pumps to the public. Due to varying factors, these companies ceased production and in the late 2000s, there were only 4–5 companies in the US. As of 2018, there are only three large companies still functioning in the USA: Medtronic Diabetes, Omnipod and Tandem. There are several more companies in Europe that are providing insulin pumps. In the future there may be additional entries into the US market from other companies. Patch pumps are of particular interest to many individuals with DM.

The use of continuous subcutaneous insulin infusion as a primary therapy for Type 2 DM patients has been investigated for the past 40 years. It has been utilized in various patient groups, including those who have newly diagnosed Type 2 DM. It is noted that individuals with Type 2 DM have poor to average control [4].

Multiple uncontrolled studies from 2008 to 2013 evaluated insulin pump therapy (CSII) in patients with Type 2 diabetes mellitus. The various studies indicated switching to CSII therapy led to improved glucose control generally, reduction in daily insulin doses compared with conventional Multiple Dose Injection therapy (MDI) and improved patient satisfaction [5]. These studies were conducted in various entities- Clinical Research Centers, Hospital outpatient clinics and small private outpatient offices.

Random Clinical Trials evaluating the efficacy of CSII therapy versus conventional MDI have been conducted and published since 1991 [6–13]. Many of these earlier studies were shorter ranging from 16 to 32 weeks and showed minimal benefit of one modality over the other.

The OpT2mise trial included a large heterogeneous population noted significant benefit compared with MDI with lower HbA1C levels, decrease in insulin requirement and no significant change in weight and no change in hypoglycemic events. This was a large scale multi center international trial which compared the efficacy of CSII therapy to intensive MDI therapy in patients who were not able to reach HbA1C goals despite intensified MDI regimens. This was a randomized parallel group study encompassing a run-in phase, 6-month randomized phase and a 6-month continuation phase. To continue in the trial a minimum of 3 measurements of glucose per day was required [14].

The study noted that CSII therapy significantly improved blood glucoses in patients when compared with MDI regimens (~ mean difference was 0.7%). There was a 20% decrease in the total insulin dose per day with little or no change in hypoglycemic events or weight gain. Additionally, these results also indicate that selection of the proper individual for CSII treatment is paramount. The study also noted that ~ 38% of patients in the CSII treatment arm had mild cognitive impairment. Patients with such impairments can successful implement CSII therapy with proper training and education.

This landmark study of CSII in Type 2 DM individuals does has some notable limitations. Patients with insulin resistance utilizing greater than 220 units per day were excluded. This is a large population which is increasing, and further large studies need to be considered. The study did not include individuals utilizing concentrated forms of insulin (U-200 and U-500).

Additionally, the study does not take in account the availability of continuous glucose monitoring and depended on serum blood glucose (SBG) monitoring. With the advent of flash glucose monitoring and advances in continuous glucose monitoring (CGM) discussed in another part of this chapter, additional studies comparing CSII and MDI in these patients may be warranted.

At present, the CSII systems available for patients with Type 2 DM include pumps with sensor combinations that have the ability to suspend delivery if the sensor notes low glucose [15].

These systems are presently the only ones approved for patients with Type 2 DM.

Future advances in CSII use for Type 2 DM could include the use of the hybrid closed loop system which now available for Type 1 DM individuals. The Medtronic hybrid closed loop system is the only one currently available. This system automatically adjusts the basal delivery every 5 minutes based on sensor readings. The system attempts to maintain glucose levels to an assigned target [16]. This form of CSII therapy functions with two different modes: Auto mode which uses an algorithm to respond to glucose levels. Manual mode is similar to previous pump-sensor combinations and requires preset basal rates by the individual in conjunction with his/her physician. Both systems still require manual meal bolus (MB) administration and manual correction for consistently elevated glucoses. Other companies are presently testing their versions of closed loop hybrid systems which may be available in the near future [17].

Patient with extreme insulin resistance have been at a disadvantage utilizing CSII therapy due to the restricted capacity of the pumps (either 180 units, 200 units, 300 units). One company in Europe has developed small insulin pumps with 500 unit and 800-unit capacity though this system is presently not available in the United States [18]. Physicians have resorted to utilizing U-500 in the pumps to decrease the frequency of site and pump changes. Several studies have noted the efficacy and improvement in quality of life with the use of U-500 in CSII therapy [19, 20]. Additional attempts to improve glucose control, quality of life, decreasing insulin requirements for Type 2 patients has led to use of so called "double pump" systems, utilizing insulin in 1 pump and pramlintide in an additional pump. Results in a small non-double-blind placebo-controlled observational study indicated a 10–20% decrease in insulin requirements, improvement in glucose control, weight loss and significant improvement in quality of life [21]. Limitations included the ability to obtain supplies for two separate pumps and utilization of pramlintide as this medication in vials was discontinued by the manufacturer at the direction of the FDA.

CSII therapy has been considered an improvement over traditional MDI therapy due to multiple factors: (1) There is predictable absorption of insulin. MDI which traditional requires injection of larger doses of insulin will form a depot and generally less efficacious in absorption and metabolic activity compared with CSII which involves smaller volumes [13]. Both the basal rate and meal bolus with CSII can be utilized with more precise insulin increments (tenths or hundredths of units). (2) Patients using CSII therapy appear to have increased satisfaction with this form of insulin therapy compared with traditional MDI injections. Based on personal observation and previous studies, patients find CSII more convenient for their lifestyle, easier to utilize after being trained and more likely to adhere to the treatment regimen. There is less likelihood of omitting (forgetting) their dose of insulin as compare with MDI. Peyrot et al. noted that patients record regular omission of insulin injections [22]. Personal observation of patients within my practice regularly indicates individuals utilizing MDI regularly admit missing meal time insulin injections. Those using CSII therapy note that since the insulin pump is attached and readily available, along with various alarm reminders missing doses is minimal. (3) The ability to download information from insulin pumps to websites (each pump has its own download capability which can cause increase work for the physician) can facilitate more efficient data collection and an ability to change the treatment regimen between patient visits.

Given the advantages of CSII therapy over MDI therapy, it would appear that CSII therapy should be considered for individuals with Type 2 DM as it is now considered for patients with Type 1 DM. However, cost effectiveness in several health systems has not been completely demonstrated. Current policies in many health systems are varied and the ability for patients to obtain access to CSII therapy may be limited.

3. Continuous glucose monitoring (CGM)

Continuous glucose monitoring or CGM was first available for research projects in the 1970s.

Miles Laboratories in the late 1970s developed the Biostator which was large, bulky and required IV access. It had little use in everyday clinical practice, due to its size, need for constant supervision, IV access and waste of blood in order to measure glucose levels [23, 24].

In 2002, the GlucoWatch Biographer was introduced. It was shaped like a watch, similar to the Apple Watches of today. It adhered to the skin and used interstitial fluid to measure glucose levels every 10 minutes for 13 hours. [25]. See **Figure 1**.

Due to its process reverse iontophoresis, the GlucoWatch had significant drawbacks. It was painful for many individuals, had accuracy issues and was difficult particularly in warmer climates with individuals sweating. The Autosensor, which was replaced every 13 hours had caused skin changes and irritation in many patients. Eventually the GlucoWatch was discontinued in late 2007. It did, however, pave the way for the CGM systems of today.

The current CGM systems use an enzymatic modality that reacts with interstitial fluid glucose and transfers it to an electrode. The electrical current that is generated is then relayed to a reader via Bluetooth wireless or an app on a smart phone which displays the results to the individual. The data can also be downloaded to a computer. Additionally, the information can be stored to the cloud and relayed to the physician or caregiver via a secure website [26].

It must be noted that interstitial glucose measurements can lag 5–15 minutes behind blood glucose measurements particularly if there is rapid variability [27, 28]. Previously, CGM systems required calibrations twice per day which introduced a perceived limitation particularly for individuals who wished to limit "finger sticks" as an incentive to move to CGM systems.

The newer versions of CGM to include the DEXCOM G6, Guardian 3 and a flash form of CGM, the FreeStyle Libre (10-day and 14-day systems) have decreased the necessity of frequent calibrations.

In recent years, there have multiple studies with CGM involving individuals with Type 2 diabetes mellitus. The focus has been efficacy, the effect of CGM

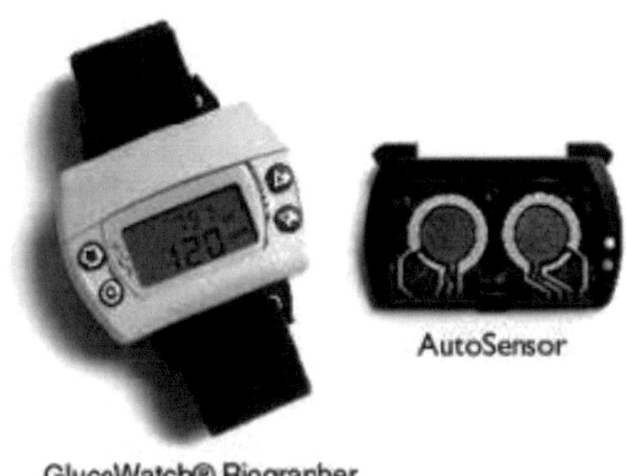

Figure 1.
GlucoWatch Biographer 2.

with regards to hypoglycemia and glucose variability [29]. A study conducted by Vigersky et al. with patients utilizing diet, lifestyle vs. other combinations of oral agent therapy with or without basal insulin noted a reduction of mean unadjusted HbA1C of 1.0% vs. 0.5% in the SMBG group at week 12 and 0.8% vs. 0.2% at week 52. This occurred without intensification of medication or an increase in hypoglycemic episodes [29]. An additional study by Fonda et al. noted even an intermittent use of CGM may be appropriate for motivating individuals or helping to avoid "burnout" [30, 31].

The DiaMonD study (Daily Injections and Continuous Glucose Monitoring in Diabetes) study was a 6-month randomized control trial that compared the effectiveness of CGM to SMBG in individuals using MDI (multiple daily injections). This included both Type 1 and Type 2 DM patients. The results of the 6-month trial for Type 2 patients was published in 2017 and noted the following: Type 2 DM individuals after 24 weeks using CGM had an average 0.8% reduction in HbA1C levels compared with baseline. Those with higher A1C levels noted the greatest reduction with a group starting with A1C levels greater than 9.0% noting an average 1.4% reduction from baseline. Those using CGM had an increase in time spent in the target range compared with the control group (those only using SMBG). The A1C reductions occurred with minimal changes in insulin doses, little or no change in regimen or addition of non-insulin medications [32].

CGM has also been useful in recognizing previously undetectable episodes of hypoglycemia. Studies conducted by Zick et al.; Pazos-Couselo et al.; Klimontov and Myakina all noted a significant higher percentage of hyperglycemic episodes observed with the use of CGM compared with SMBG use.

The use of CGM particularly in older individuals utilizing insulin therapy has noted significantly higher incidences of nocturnal hypoglycemia compared with those utilizing only CGM. This indicates that CGM can be useful in high-risk Type 2 DM populations such as the elderly, those with special needs and individuals that have difficulty utilizing HGM such as severe arthritic conditions, vascular issues, etc. [33–36].

CGM is also a tool to assess glucose variability. This has become important in outcome measurements recently in addition to the standard A1C levels. The INITIATION study which tested an insulin initiation algorithm in Type 2 DM patients used CGM in 78 patients who were followed for 24 weeks. The results noted that insulin initiation reduced hyperglycemia but not glucose variability [37, 38]. The FLAT-SUGAR study which randomized 102 patients who were on metformin and basal/bolus insulin to either maintenance with basal/bolus therapy for changing the basal insulin to GLP-1 therapy. The drug used with this study of 26 weeks was exenatide BID. Using CGM it was noted that the GLP-1 group had lower variability of glucose as measured by the coefficient of variation. Of note with this study, A1C levels or episodes of hypoglycemia did note change significantly between the treatment groups [39–41].

These studies and others both past and presently being conducted have shown the CGM use in patients with Type 2 DM can improve A1C levels, detect risk of hypoglycemia which is not clinically apparent, particularly nocturnally and may be able to assess and address glucose variability.

There are two forms of CGM presently available for use in clinical practice: (1) Professional CGM and (2) Personal CMG. Professional CGM is placed in the physician office and does not require the patient to obtain or purchase a system. It is a blinded system in many instances, that is, the patient has no access to the results immediately and must wait for the CGM to be downloaded in the physician's office, analyzed and then informed of the results. These systems can be worn for 3, 7 or 14 days, though generally the 7- or 14-day systems are more popular today. The systems available today in the United States for professional use are: the DEXCOM Professional system, the FreeStyle Libre Pro system, Medtronic iPro 2 system. Most of these systems do require additional calibration. Once the study is completed, the data is downloaded to either the cloud or a specific program on the computer and then can be reviewed by the physician or allied health provider in conjunction with the physician and then shared with the patient. The blinded system can be helpful in regards that the patient is not responding during the time of the study but continuing their usual habits to include diet, activity and medications. Reimbursement for use of Professional CGM has improved over the past several years particularly in the United States. Requirements as the reporting of CGM results can vary among the different health plans which can lead to limitations in its use.

Personal CGM consists of an individual obtaining a system which is unblinded and provides blood glucoses every 5+ minutes for DEXCOM and Guardian 3 systems. These systems are placed subcutaneously and have alarms with notify the patient when certain patterns or thresholds are detected. There are multiple threshold alarms, rate of change alarms, predictive alarms. Predictive alarms are useful in that it permits the individual to take preventative action rather than corrective action. However, the downside of these alarms is that there can be false positives and false negatives. This can lead to so-called "alarm fatigue" [42]. Individuals will in many instances either ignore or silence the systems due to the multitude of alarms. In some cases, they will abandon CGM altogether. The DEXCOM G5–6 system is the only CGM device at present that is approved by the FDA for a non-adjunctive indication. It can be considered a therapeutic CGM, allowing individuals and physicians to modify therapy based solely on the readings and trends.

The FreeStyle Libre system utilizes a flash monitoring system. It is placed like the other CGM systems subcutaneously but provides glucose results when the CGM is scanned. Thus, the results are intermittent depending on the frequency of scanning by the patient [43]. The newest of the FreeStyle Libre systems, the 14-day unit improves over the older 10-day system with a 1-hour warm up period compared with 12 hours. Several randomized controlled trails note that the use of flash CGM with the Libre system reduced hypoglycemia, increased the time in target range and reduced glucose variability [44, 45] Studies and personal observation have also shown higher device utilization. This may be due to the simplicity of application and ease of use. The use of this system in increasing and may prove to be an asset particularly in individuals who may not need the sophistication of the more complex CGM system but want the benefit of CGM and not have to consistently perform SMBG or finger sticks.

Additional studies in Europe have shown the cost effectiveness of CGM in the management of patients with Type 2 DM receiving intensive MDI regimens and also improvement in the detection and avoidance of hypoglycemia in individuals with Type 2 DM [46, 47].

Another technological advance in CGM has been the development and approval of the implantable CGM system by Senseonics called the Eversense System. The system consists of an implantable cylindrical sensor 3.5 mm × 18.3 mm in size. This is implanted by the physician every 90 days in the upper arm area under the skin. When the system in activated, it measures interstitial glucose levels every 5 minutes. The data is transferred to a battery powered transmitter that is worn externally over the sensor. The external transmitter also provides alerts similar to other CGM systems for impending hypo or hyperglycemia. The transmitter needs to be recharged for ~15 minutes every other day. The sensor is explanted, and a new sensor implanted every 90 days. A 180-day sensor is being developed for the future.

Several studies have shown the accuracy and acceptability of an implantable glucose sensor. The PRECISE and PRECISE II studies noted that the Eversense system was safe and provided accurate glucose results during the 90-day sensor life [48, 49]. An additional study in the UK and Germany comprising a subgroup of individuals in the PRECISE trial who were administered quantitative psychosocial assessments that included the Diabetes Distress Scale (DDS), CGM Impact Scale and a bespoke device satisfaction questionnaire. The results of the sub study indicated that an implantable CGM was acceptable to most of the participants and the majority of users both first time to CGM or previous CGM users would continue to use an implantable CGM to manage their glucoses and DM more effectively [50].

As the accuracy of CGM improves, particularly in the hypoglycemia range, the acceptance should also increase. However, at this time, CGM still does not, in the eyes of the regulatory agencies substitute fully for conventional SBGM. With continued development and use, it appears that eventually CGM, with or without CSII therapy will become the “standard of care” for both Type 1 and Type 2 diabetes mellitus.

4. Smart pen systems

Most individuals with DM, particularly Type 2 DM, who utilize insulin therapy are using insulin pen systems to deliver their daily insulin dose. Previous administration of insulin via syringe and vial has been difficult to administer and master. Additionally, accuracy of dose has been questioned. Insulin pens are one of the most widely used devices worldwide in DM treatment and care [51].

A recent review of the literature and meta-analysis noted that insulin pen devices noted improvement in patient adherence and persistence with their treatment regimen. Hypoglycemia was noted to be reduced, with a possible improvement in dose accuracy in pen devices. However, these studies were limited, and the authors of the meta-analysis recommended additional larger scale studies [52].

Additionally, there is the issue of documentation of insulin doses. Many patients do not record the time and dose of insulin consistently. Many will state that they took their insulin with meals, nighttime, for correction of their glucose, etc. but will not be able to provide accurate documentation. Therefore, this can be a significant barrier to glycemic control. Guidelines developed by various organizations make no mention of the need to record insulin dose administered and timing of injection whether the patient uses pen or syringe/vial.

In December 2017, the FDA approved the first smart pen system in the US. This insulin pen system records the dose of insulin and time of injection and transmits the data via Bluetooth to a mobile application that is downloaded on the patient’s smart phone. The mobile app has the capability of dose calculation and less than whole number units which conventional insulin pens are not able to deliver.

It can also inform the individual how much insulin is on board (IOB) similar to CSII devices. This data is stored on the individuals’ smart phone and can be brought easily to the clinical visit for analysis by the physician/health care provider.

There may an additional entry in this area. Bigfoot Biomedical is developing an insulin smart pen that will connect to the FreeStyle Libre system. It will be controlled with a mobile app and hopefully adjust long and short acting insulin doses without manual input [53].

The benefits of a smart pen system in the treatment of individuals with DM can be summarized as follows:

1. Improvement in poor adherence to the treatment regimen and omission of insulin doses.

Having the data readily available and reminders on their phone can provide an extra incentive to be more compliant with their regimen.

2. Improvement with the risk of insulin dose errors. Access to dosing and timing of insulin can facilitate more accurate doses and limit the risk of accidental overdose or under dosing.

This being a relatively new technology, these devices will need to demonstrate improvement in clinical and QOL (Quality of Life) outcomes, cost effectiveness, ease of training and use. However, many of the technologies discussed above have underwent the same scrutiny. The issue of cybersecurity as with any connected DM devices will need to be resolved to maintain patient confidentiality and integrity of the data. Smart pens may be an alternative to individuals who do not want CSII therapy for a multitude of reasons but would like to intensify their regimen and have access to appropriate dosing and timing of insulin to improve their glucose control.

5. Mobile and computer applications (apps)

Data Management software for diabetes has been available since the late 1980s to early 1990s. However, acceptance and adoption by both patients and physicians has been slow. The issues have been the ability to download or upload data with each device having its own set of software and cable connections. In many cases, physician offices had upwards of 6–10 different connections to obtain data from SMBG meters and other devices.

Over the past two decades, a number of innovations were developed that "streamlined" the ability to obtain data from patient devices. There has been an improvement in device connectivity with most devices now able to utilize Bluetooth technology thus eliminating the need for multiple cables or hubs. Additionally, smartphone technology has decreased the cost and complexity of data sharing. The use of automated uploads from devices to the "cloud" has allowed both patient and physician to have almost real-time access to data [53].

Proprietary cloud data platforms from multiple device manufacturers have been able to provide secure data and have developed common formats, easing the burden on physicians and their offices to maintain multiple programs. Also, many of the device companies, including those manufacturing SMBG devices have developed complex reporting capabilities that have been designated as Ambulatory Glucose Reports or Profiles.

The multitude of apps for the patient with DM has led to concerns of quality and safety. Apps available at both the Google Play store and Apple App Store may little or no oversight. A recent study in 2016 found that the majority of apps from the Google Play store did not meet the minimum requirements or did not work appropriately [54, 56] Additional studies are needed to fully investigate the efficacy and utility of mobile applications with regard to the treatment of individuals with Type 2 DM.

Another approach is to combine the mobile application, the cloud with a remote coaching system. Studies are now ongoing to assess the effect of individuals using a smart phone-based glucose monitoring system which automatically moves data to a secure cloud-based site [55]. A designated "diabetes coach" which is a health care provider (RN, NP or physician) then reviews the data several times per week and remotely connects with the patient to provide recommendations or discussion. Results are pending in these studies and hopefully preliminary results will be available in 2019. (Personal Observation).

The use of Artificial Intelligence (AI) in the treatment of patients with Diabetes is emerging and advancing at significant pace. Multiple programs are being developed to improve adherence and personalize the individual's regimen. Studies are ongoing to determine whether pattern recognition and the ability of machine learning can provide the patient with diabetes mellitus a unique, individualize model which is automated and can assist with predictions and decisions. At this time, AI cannot and does not substitute for patient – physician interaction and communication.

6. Conclusion

This chapter attempted to briefly outline the technological advances in the treatment of Type 2 diabetes mellitus. It is noted the technology has improved the quality of life, blood glucose control and possibly decreased the risk of complications. However, it must be pointed out to the reader that technology, no matter how advanced, does not substitute for personal interaction with patients. The ability to know your patient, his/her lifestyle, stressors, etc. plays an important role in designing the proper treatment regimen. Continued advances in technology will in the future make the physician/healthcare provider and the patient's ability to control his/her blood glucoses less complicated but ultimately the decisions to maintain diet, exercise, monitoring of glucoses remains with the individual.

Conflicts of interest

The author notes that he is a member of the DSMB and CEC for Medtronic Diabetes and serves on the Speaker's Bureau for Sanofi and Astra Zeneca.

Notes/thanks/other declarations

The author wishes to thank his wife for assisting in the research for this chapter and his associate and staff for permitting him to devote extra time from the practice to complete this endeavor.

Author details

Alan B. Schorr[1,2]

1 Chairman Department of Medicine, Saint Mary Medical Center, USA

2 Division Head Endocrinology, Saint Mary Medical Center, USA

*Address all correspondence to: abs@sugardoc.com

References

[1] Taylor R. Pathogenesis of type 2 diabetes: Tracing the reverse route from cure to cause. Diabetologia. 2008;**51**:1781-1789

[2] Despres JP, Poirier P. Diabetes: Looking back at a look AHEAD-giving lifestyle a chance. Nature Reviews Cardiology. 2013;**10**:184-186

[3] Heinemann L, Flemming GA, Petrie JR, Holl RW, Bergenstal RM, Peters AL. Insulin pump risks and benefits: A clinical appraisal of pump safety standards, adverse event reporting and research needs. Diabetes Care. 2015;**38**(4):716-722. DOI: 10.2337/dc15-0168

[4] Pickup JC. Insulin pump therapy for type 2 diabetes mellitus. Nature Reviews. Endocrinology. 2014;**10**: 647-649. DOI: 10.1038/nendo.2014.142

[5] Gentry CK, Cross LB, Gross BN, McFarland MD, Besterman WH. Retrospective analysis and patient satisfaction assessment of insulin pump therapy in patients with type 2 diabetes. Southern Medical Journal. 2011;**104**(1):24-28

[6] Goa G-Q, Heng X-Y, Y-l W, et al. Comparison of continuous subcutaneous insulin infusion and insulin glargine based multiple daily insulin aspart injections with preferential adjustment of basal insulin in patients with type 2 diabetes. Experimental and Therapeutic Medicine. 2014;**8**(4):1191-1196

[7] Wolf-McDonagh P, Kaufmann J, Foreman S, Wisotsky S, Wisotsky JAJA, Wexler C. Using insulin pump therapy in poorly controlled type 2 diabetes. The Diabetes Educator;**36**(4):657-665

[8] Landau Z, Raz I, Weinstein J, Bar-Dayan CA. The role of insulin pump therapy for type 2 diabetes mellitus. Diabetes/Metabolism Research and Reviews. 2017;**33**:e2822. DOI: 10.1002/dmrr.2822

[9] Raskin P, Bode BW, Marks JB, et al. Continuous subcutaneous insulin infusion and multiple daily injection therapy are equally effective in type 2 diabetes: A randomized parallel-group, 24-week study. Diabetes Care. 2003;**26**(9):2598-2603

[10] Wainstein J, Metzger M, Boaz M, et al. Insulin pump therapy vs. multiple daily injections in obese type 2 diabetic patients. Diabetic Medicine. 2005;**22**(8):1037-1046

[11] Parkner T, Laursen T, Vestergard ET, et al. Insulin and glucose profiled during continuous subcutaneous insulin infusion compared with injection of a long acting insulin in type 2 diabetes. Diabetic Medicine. 2008;**25**(5):585-591

[12] Weng J, Li Y, Xu W, et al. Short-term intensive therapy in newly diagnosed type 2 diabetes partially restores both insulin sensitivity and beta cell function in subjects with long term remission. Diabetes Care. 2011;**34**(8):1848-1853

[13] Herman WH, Ilag LI, Johnson SI, et al. A clinical trial of continuous subcutaneous insulin infusion versus multiple daily injections in older adults with type 2 diabetes. Diabetes Care. 2005;**28**(7):1568-1573

[14] Reznik Y, Cohen O, Aronson R, Ignacio C, Runzis S, Castaneda J, et al. Insulin pump treatment compared with multiple daily injections for treatment of type 2 diabetes (OpT2mise): A randomized open-label controlled trial. Lancet. 2014;**384**:1265-1272. DOI: 10.1016/S0140-6736(14)61037-0

[15] Medtronic: Innovation Milestones. 2018. Available from: https://www.

medtronicdiabetes.com/about-medtronic-innovation.milestone-timeline [Accessed: r 12-12-2018]

[16] Weaver KW, Hirsch IB. The hybrid closed-loop system: Evolutions and practical applications. Diabetes Technology & Therapeutics. 2018;**20**(Suppl 2):S2-S16. DOI: 10.1089/dia.2018.0091

[17] Trevitt S, Simpson S, Wood A. Artificial pancreas device systems for the closed loop control of type 1 diabetes: What systems are in development. Journal of Diabetes Science and Technology. 2016;**10**:714-723. DOI: 10.1177/1932296815617968

[18] Debiotech: Jewel Insulin Pump. Available from: https://www.debiotech.com/page/index.php?page=product_01&id=1&id_prod=40 [Accessed: 14-12-2018]

[19] Reutrakul S, Wroblewski K, Brown RL. Clinical use of U-500 regular insulin: Review and meta-analysis. Journal of Diabetes Science and Technology. 2012;**6**:412-420

[20] Lane WS, Weinrib SL, Rappaport JM, Hale CB, Farmer LK, Lane RS. The effect of long-term use of U-500 via continuous subcutaneous infusion on durability of glycemic control and weight in obese, insulin-resistance patients with type 2 diabetes. Endocrine Practice. 2012;**27**:1-18

[21] Schorr AB, Ofan R. Simultaneous use of two external subcutaneous pumps delivering insulin and SYMLIN: Use of a double-pump system. Journal of Diabetes Science and Technology. 2012;**6**:1507-1508

[22] Peyrot M, Rubin R. Validity and reliability of an instrument for assessing health-related quality of life and treatment preferences-the insulin delivery system rating questionnaire. Diabetes Care;**28**(1):33-39

[23] Clarke SF, Foster JR. A history of blood glucoses meters and their role in self-monitoring of diabetes mellitus. British Journal of Biomedical Science. 2012;**69**:83-93

[24] Skyler JS. CGM-a technology in evolution. Diabetes Technology & Therapeutics. 2009;**11**:63-64

[25] The Diabetes Research in Children Network (DirecNet) Study Group. A randomized multicenter trial comparing the GlucoWatch Biographer with standard glucose monitoring in children with type 1 diabetes. Diabetes Care. 2005;**28**:1101-1106

[26] Klonoff DC, Ahn D, Drincic A. Continuous glucose monitoring: A review of the technology and clinical use. Diabetes Research and Clinical Practice. 2017;**133**:178-192. DOI: 10.1016/j.diabres.2017.08.005

[27] Rebel A, Rice MA, Fahy BG. Accuracy or point-of-care glucose measurements. Journal of Diabetes Science and Technology. 2012;**6**(2):396-411

[28] Vaddiraju S et al. Technologies for continuous glucose monitoring: Current problems and future promises. Journal of Diabetes Science and Technology. 2010;**4**(6):1540-1562

[29] Carlson AL, Mullen DM, Bergenstal RM. Clinical use of continuous glucose monitoring in adults with type 2 diabetes. Diabetes Technology & Therapeutics. 2017;**19**(Suppl 2):s-4-s-11. DOI: 10.1089/dia.2017.0024

[30] Vigersky RA, Fonda SJ, Chellappa M, et al. Short and long-term effects of real-time continuous glucose monitoring in patients with type 2 diabetes. Diabetes Care. 2012;**35**:32-38

[31] Sj F, Graham C, Munakata J, et al. The cost effectiveness of real-time continuous glucose monitoring

(RT-CGM) in type 2 diabetes. Journal of Diabetes Science and Technology. 2016;**10**:898-904. DOI: 10.1177/1932296816628547

[32] Beck RW, Riddlesworth TD, Ruedy K, Ahmann A, Haller S, Kruger D, et al. Continuous glucose monitoring versus usual Care in Patients with type 2 diabetes receiving multiple daily injections – A randomized Trial. Annals of Internal Medicine. 2017;**167**(6):365-374. DOI: 10.7326/M16-2855

[33] Zick R, Peterson B, Richter M, Haug C. Comparison of continuous blood glucose measurement with conventional documentation of hypoglycemia in patients with type 2 diabetes on multiple daily insulin injection therapy. Diabetes Technology & Therapeutics. 2007;**9**:483-492

[34] Pazos-Couselo M, Garcia-Lopez JM, Gonzalez-Rodriquez M, et al. High incidence of hypoglycemia in stable insulin treated type 2 diabetes mellitus: Continuous glucose monitoring vs. self-monitored blood glucose. Observational prospective study. Canadian Journal of Diabetes. 2015;**39**:428-433. DOI: doi.org/10.1016/j.jcjd.2015.05.007

[35] Klimontov VV, Myakina NE. Glucose variability indices predict the episodes of nocturnal hypoglycemia in elderly type 2 diabetic patients treated with insulin. Diabetes and Metabolic Syndrome: Clinical Research and Reviews. 2017;**11**:119-124

[36] Gomez AM, Umpierrez GE, Munoz OM, et al. Continuous glucose monitoring vs. capillary point-of-care testing for inpatient glycemic control in type 2 diabetes patients hospitalized in the general ward and treated with basal-bolus insulin regimen. Journal of Diabetes Science and Technology. 2016;**10**:325-329. DOI: 10.1177/1932296815602905

[37] Kovatchev B, Cobelli C. Glucose variability: Timing, risk analysis, and relationship to hypoglycemia in diabetes. Diabetes Care. 2016;**39**: 502-510. DOI: 10.2337/dc15-2035

[38] Manski-Nankervis J-A, Furler J, Blackberry I, et al. Roles and relationships between health professional involved in insulin initiation for people with type 2 diabetes in the general practice setting: A qualitative study drawing on relational coordination theory. BMC Family Practice. 2014;**15**:20

[39] Prostfield Jl et al. Flat Sugar Trial Investigators: Glucose variability in a 26-week randomized comparison of mealtime treatment with rapid-acting insulin versus GLP-1 agonist in participants with type 2 diabetes at high cardiovascular risk. Diabetes Care. 2016;**39**:973-981. DOI: 10.2337/dc15-2782

[40] Xu F, Zhao L-H, Su J-B, et al. The relationship between glycemic variability and diabetic neuropathy in type 2 diabetes with well controlled HbA1c. Diabetology & Metabolic Syndrome. 2014;**6**:139

[41] Sartore G, Chilelli NC, Burlina S, Lapolla A. Association between glucose variability as assessed by continuous glucose monitoring (CGM) and diabetic retinopathy in type 1 and type 2 diabetes. Acta Diabetologica. 2013;**50**:437-442

[42] Shivers JP et al. "Turn it off!"; diabetes device alarm fatigue considerations for the present and the future. Journal of Diabetes Science and Technology. 2013;7(3):789-794

[43] Kudva YC, Ahmann AJ, Bergenstal RM, Gavin JR III, Kruger DF, Midyett LK, et al. Approach to using trend arrows in the FreeStyle Libre flash glucose monitoring Systems in Adults. Journal of the Endocrine Society.

2018;**2**(12):1320-1337. DOI: 10.1210/js.2018-00294

[44] Bolinder J, Antuna R, Geelhowed-Duijvestijn P, Kroder J, Weitgasser R. Novel glucose-sensing technology and hypoglycaemia in type 1 diabetes. A multicenter, non-masked randomized controlled trial. Lancet;**388**(10057):2254-2263. DOI: 10.1016/S0140-6736(16)31535-5

[45] Haak T, Hanaire H, Ajjan R, Hermanns N, Riveline JP, Rayman G. Flash glucose-sensing technology as a replacement for blood glucose monitoring for the management of insulin-treated type 2 diabetes: A multicenter open-label randomized controlled trial. Diabetes Therapy. 2017;**8**(1):55-73. DOI: 10.1007/s13300-016-0223-6

[46] Bilir SP, Hellmund R, Wehler E, Li H, Munakata J, Lamotte M. The cost-effectiveness of flash glucose monitoring system for management of patients with type 2 diabetes receiving intensive insulin treatment in Sweden. European Endocrinology. 2018;**14**(2):80-85. DOI: 10.17925/EE.2018.14.2.80

[47] Adolfsson P, Rentoul D, Klinkenbiji PCG. Hypoglycemia remains the key obstacle to optimal Glycemic control-continuous glucose monitoring is the solution. European Endocrinology. 2018;**14**(2):50-56. DOI: 10.17925/EE.2018.14.2.50

[48] Kropff J, Choudhary P, Neupane S, Barnard K, Bain S, Kapitza C, et al. Accuracy and longevity of an implantable continuous glucose sensor in the PRECISE study: A 180-day, prospective, Multicenter, pivotal Trial. Diabetes Care. 2017;**40**:1-6. DOI: 10.2337/dc16-1525

[49] Christianson MP, Klaff LJ, Brazg R, Chang AR, Levey CJ, Lam D, et al. A prospective Multicenter evaluation of the accuracy of a novel implanted continuous glucose sensor: PRECISE II. Diabetes Technology & Therapeutics. 2018;**20**(3):1-10. DOI: 10.1089/dia.2017.0142

[50] Barnard KD, Kropff J, Choudhary P, Neuopane S, Bain SC, Kapitza C, et al. Acceptability of implantable continuous glucose monitoring sensor. Journal of Diabetes Science and Technology. 2017;**12**(3):634-638. DOI: 10.1177/1932296817735123

[51] Klonoff DC, Kerr D. Smart pens will improve insulin therapy. Journal of Diabetes Science and Technology. 2018;**12**(3):551-553. DOI: 10.1177/1932296818759845

[52] Lasalva P, Barahona-Correa J, Romero-Alvernia DM, Gil-Tomayo S, Castaneda-Cardona C, Bayona JG, et al. Pen devices for insulin self administration compared with needle and vial: Systematic review of the literature and meta-analysis. Journal of Diabetes Science and Technology. 2106;**10**(4):959-966. DOI: 10.1177/1932296816633721

[53] Baily TS, Walsh J, Stone JY. Emerging technologies for diabetes care. Diabetes Technology & Therapeutics. 2018;**20**(s2):78-84. DOI: 10.1089/dia.2018.0115

[54] Coughlin SS. Mobile technology for self-monitoring of blood glucose among patients with type 2 diabetes mellitus. mHealth. 2017;**3**:47-50. DOI: 10.21037/mhealth.2017.10.03

[55] Brzan PP, Rotman E, Pajnkihar M, et al. Mobile applications for control and self-management of diabetes; a systematic review. Journal of Medical Systems. 2016;**40**:210. DOI: 10.1007/s10916-016-0564-8

[56] Huang Z, Soljak M, Boehm BO, Car J. Clinical relevance of smartphone apps for diabetes management: A global overview. Diabetes/Metabolism Research and Reviews. 2018;**34**:e2990. DOI: 10.1002/dmrr.2990

Chapter 7

Cyber-Physical System for Management and Self-Management of Cardiometabolic Health

Zsolt Peter Ori

Abstract

We want to demonstrate the feasibility of the concept of a cyber-physical system (CPS) by showing good correlation of insulin resistance by HOMA-IR with changes of state variables (SVs) such as R-ratio, Rw-ratio, calculated 24 h nonprotein respiratory quotient, and fat-burning fraction from serial measurements of weight and fat mass. We utilize principles of indirect calorimetry. We calculate SVs from published data of an energy perturbation study. We perform correlation analysis between changes of insulin resistance measured with HOMA-IR and selected SVs. The result of this correlation analysis confirms a highly significant correlation between HOMA-IR and the selected SVs. The implication of these results is that CPS is a suitable concept to indirectly measure and predict the otherwise very-difficult- or impossible-to-measure slow changes of SVs and capture them for the first time noninvasively. Serial fat and weight measurements and energy calculations can help unmask changes of insulin resistance in response to user's diet and exercise habits, creating the necessary environment to measure metabolic flexibility. Further, CPS has the potential to estimate cardiorespiratory fitness by indirectly estimating maximum oxygen uptake from measuring heart rate reserve, heart rate variability, and pulse oximetry changes with exercise.

Keywords: energy metabolism, metabolic profile, insulin resistance, metabolic monitoring, cardiometabolic health, self-management

1. Introduction

This book chapter introduces to practicing physicians the framework of our cyber-physical system (CPS) for management and self-management of cardiometabolic health. The hypothesis here is that cardiometabolic functions relevant to cardiovascular disease (CVD) mortality including insulin resistance can be tracked and predicted from measuring physical activity, heart rate, and pulse oximetry by a smart watch and from serial weight and fat weight measurements obtained from a bioimpedance fat scale. CPS serves the need for individualized precision methods to gauge cardiometabolic health with metrics/trajectories and predict slow changes of cardiometabolic health in health as well as in disease. There is a need to provide this information as a feedback to patients and their care team to facilitate prevention and treatment of chronic noncommunicable disease, improve rehabilitation after acute cardiovascular illness, and facilitate needed behavior change for cardiometabolic risk reduction to improve cardiovascular as well as all-cause mortality. Computer-generated feedback may provide a framework for automation and self-improvement to meet daily goals of therapeutic efforts.

Based on our research in systems biology, a cyber-physical system (CPS) can be construed for noninvasively tracking, drawing trajectories, and indirectly measuring daily changes and predict the otherwise very-difficult- or impossible-to-measure slow changes of the daily *s*tate *v*ariables (SVs) of the metabolism and capture them for the first time noninvasively in freely moving humans in their natural environment outside of a metabolic laboratory setting.

Components of CPS are (A) a management software tool (MST); (B) a metabolic health monitor (MHM) app; (C) software on MHM capturing biometric signals from sensors of heart rate, physical activity, and pulse oximetry from a smart watch; and (D) software on MHM capturing biometric signals related to body composition and hydration status from Ori Diagnostic Instruments' (ODI) patented apparatus for impedance spectroscopy. MHM is running ODI's proprietary self-adaptive individualized stochastic mathematical model of the human energy metabolism (SAM-HEM) [1–3] via cloud computing. Based on our published simulation studies, SAM-HEM is a suitable concept to capture daily changes of the following SVs: weight; fat mass; lean mass; protein mass; intracellular water mass; extracellular water mass; utilized macronutrient intake and substrate oxidation of carbohydrate, fat, protein; and the R-ratio (ratio of the daily lean mass change velocity divided by the daily fat mass change velocity) which could be used as a surrogate marker for insulin resistance. SAM-HEM is a self-learning algorithm with daily updates using the minimal variance Kalman filter/predictor to arrive at the best metabolic model fitting to the available measured data. The trajectories of SVs are displayed on MHM and MST with errors of calculations allowing for analysis of past events, tracking current metabolic events real time, predicting metabolic changes in the future, and supporting self-management as well as guided therapies. We envision also that the same smart watch can provide sufficient information to track cardiorespiratory fitness by estimated maximum oxygen uptake. Our innovation is to merge the assessment of metabolic fitness/flexibility measurements with the assessment of cardiorespiratory fitness and realize CPS to improve cardiometabolic health.

The challenges ahead are the following: The prevalence of obesity and type 2 diabetes (T2D) is ranked the highest in the USA and Mexico in the American continent [4]. The proportion of the population with abnormal glucose tolerance is 52.4% for the USA (14.4% T2D, 38% prediabetes) [5] and 33.5% for Mexico (14.1% T2D, 19.1% prediabetes) [6].

Central to our mission in primary care is to fight the burden of noncommunicable chronic diseases including the most prominent one, cardiovascular disease (CVD). CVD is substantially higher in individuals with unhealthy lifestyle characteristics, including obesity, prediabetes, diabetes, insulin resistance, metabolic syndrome, physical inactivity, poor diet, and cigarette smoking [7]. In forging the battle against these problems, I see the following paramount problems:

1. There is a certain degree of fatigue toward "dieting," "weight loss," and hearing the word "obese." According to a recent survey [8], many sufferers of obesity wanted to become "healthy" so they could be "fit" and "strong" and expressed the wish for general health.

2. The problem with targeting weight loss only is that it does not distinguish between the loss of adipose and lean tissues. Further, it intuitively contradicts

the notion of the obesity paradox, i.e., increased BMI is associated with increased survival and reduced mortality among patients with cardiovascular risk [9]. A mortality study in adults showed that normal weight at the time of incident diabetes had higher mortality than adults who are overweight or obese [9, 10]. This apparent obesity paradox is best explained by insulin resistance which is the primary underlying factor in cardiovascular disease. Fat mass itself and insulin sensitivity (reciprocal of insulin resistance) may be the decisive link between mortality and weight status [10]. Moreover, a more recent study [11] confirms what most clinicians have felt for a long time that obesity or excess fat mass with associated insulin resistance is directly associated with shorter longevity and significantly increased risk of cardiovascular morbidity and mortality [11]. Furthermore, when a surrogate index of insulin resistance such as waist circumference is used to predict mortality, an elevated waistline was strongly predictive of an increased mortality rate among patients with cardiovascular disease [12], and it is an independent risk factor for CVD mortality [13].

3. Clearly, there is a need for healthy lifestyle interventions using self-management along with support team approach to prevent and treat noncommunicable diseases linked to overweight and obesity [14] to achieve cardiorespiratory fitness along with metabolic health with lowest possible insulin resistance. Effective programs and technology tools together are needed to support behavior change approaches toward healthy lifestyle. Recently, behavior change strategies have emphasized the need for feedback loops for self-directed behavior modification [15]. However, there is a paucity of personalized, time-adjusted, dynamic interventions supporting feedback control for health behavior interventions [16]. There is a needed tool to observe the slow changes of cardiovascular fitness and metabolic health metrics closely as a feedback of information for patient and primary care provider to facilitate self-directed behavior change [3] as well as for guided therapy by the healthy lifestyle team. The hurdles to develop such behavior change models with dynamic feedback loops and corresponding supportive technology tools are (A) the lack of gold standard measures for important behavior constructs, (B) tools allowing for planning and executing dynamic changes of behavior, (C) a dynamic behavior change model using self-directed behavioral change strategies, and (D) outcome measures for optimization [3, 16].

Given the pandemic of overweight and obesity involving 1.9 billion people worldwide according to the World Health Organization, new and fresh ideas and approaches are needed. One of the goals of the current article is to introduce to researchers and clinicians a widely applicable toolset which could unleash the potential of the modern Digital Era and tackle the extraordinary burden of insulin resistance, obesity, prediabetes, metabolic syndrome, and type 2 diabetes on humanity. In this article, inspirations were taken from thoughts and works of giant and prodigious scientists of the twentieth century, the unbelievably huge potential of smartphone technologies, combined with the tremendous power of human networking through the Internet. With the current novel framework, we strive to use the minimum set of assumptions about the process and measurement.

Eugene Wigner (1902–1995) stated that there is a "miracle of the appropriateness of the language of mathematics for the formulation of the laws of physics" ... which may appear to us with "unreasonable efficiency." The inspiration here is, why not use mathematical tools for the formulation of the applicable laws to the human energy metabolism such as the first and second laws of the thermodynamics when considering, for example, the fat balance, i.e., fat in minus fat out? Though indirect calorimetry already makes reference to these laws, the indirect calorimetry technology use is intricately connected to respiratory gas exchange measurements which are difficult to do with the daily routine of life. However, mathematical models can be created with input variables with easier realization in daily life such as weight and fat weight measurement with bioimpedance fat scale. Further, appropriately built mathematical models can provide indirect measurements of difficult-to-measure variables of the human energy metabolism like fat versus carbohydrate oxidation rate or changes of insulin resistance [1–3] and provide a solution to gain a special quantified insight into the fat and the entire energy metabolism. Currently, the computational model of the human energy metabolism (CM-HEM) [17] and its improved version [18] is considered the most complete. CM-HEM uses the three compartmental partitioning of the entire energy flow, centered around the major macronutrient energy stores: glycogen G, fat F, and protein P. Hall was able to test his model and found satisfactory agreement between the model predictions and the measured group averaged data from the Minnesota Study [17], as well as 50 other studies [18]. Although CM-HEM behaves appropriately for different groups of subjects, it is presently unclear whether individual subject responses can be predicted [19], and CM-HEM may be limited in its ability to provide precise information on an individual basis [19]. Further, CM-HEM uses food intake as an input rather than an output variable, and it would be particularly interesting to determine utilized food intake from body composition changes [19]. CM-HEM is neither linear nor recursive nor individualized to a particular subject, and therefore, it is not suited to performing recursive parameter identification of the human energy metabolism, nor is it able to perform inverse calculation of utilized energy intake. Further, insulin resistance is not considered in CM-HEM when in fact insulin resistance plays a crucial role influencing fat and carbohydrate oxidation rates and the entire dynamic of body composition change [1–3]. Obviously, individualized models are needed which can be tied to easily measurable input variables such as weight and fat weight and provide insight into the fat and nonfat energy balance and change of insulin resistance.

A second insightful guidance to our approach comes from John von Neumann (1903–1957) for the fight against insulin resistance. During his time, he foresaw already that "science, as well as technology, will in the near and in the farther future increasingly turn to problems of structure, organization, information, and control." This raises the question, why not use Neumann's self-organization and system theory ideas to control and prevent insulin resistance and obesity? In this regard using certain universal principles for energy calculation, such as the principle of "least action/ stationary action," for example, in Lagrangian and Hamiltonian mechanics, can be instrumental in setting up suitable control equations or functionals, such as the Hamilton-Jacobi-Bellman equation in control theory for dynamic optimized control [20]. This Hamilton-Jacobi-Bellman equation can allow for dynamic optimization of the energy system to achieve the desired state in the shortest possible time with minimized efforts.

The third inspirational insight comes from Rudolf E. Kálmán (1930–2016) and his invention of the "Kalman filter." This is briefly a statistical tool with tremendously widely used successful applications to control a vast array of consumer, health, commercial, and defense products. According to Grewal [21], the Kalman Filter is possibly the greatest discovery in the twentieth century and made the moon landing among others possible. This raises the question, why not use the Kalman filter to estimate and predict fat mass change? A potential application of Kalman's minimum variance estimator and predictor could be twofold: (1) Updating the a priori estimation equations for the measurement variables (weight, fat weight) with a posteriori results and (2) providing a posteriori estimation for the process variables such as lean mass L, glycogen mass G, fat mass F, protein P, intracellular water mass ICW, and extracellular water mass ECW. This will realize a dynamic state-space modeling connecting the measured variables with the process variables, never losing the measured reality and keeping full statistical knowledge about confidence intervals and other statistical properties of results. The beauty of the Kalman estimators is that they operate also as a predictor when no updated measurements are provided.

Central to the development of the noninvasive metrics for the human energy metabolism is to have a novel metric for insulin resistance from energy flow point of view through the body. Insulin resistance is related to ectopic fat accumulation and reduced capacity of fat oxidation and inflexibility in regulating fat oxidation combined with the increased propensity of glucose oxidation and glucose-induced suppression of fat oxidation [22]. Experimental weight perturbation showed concordant changes of the glucose vs. fat oxidation fraction in skeletal muscle [23]. The correlation between BMI/weight/body composition and insulin resistance measured, for example, with Homeostatic Model Assessment of Insulin Resistance (HOMA-IR), is well documented in the medical literature [24, 25]. It is increasingly recognized also that there is a dynamic correlation between changes of weight, fat weight, and insulin sensitivity/resistance changes. Building on the above observations and reviewing energy perturbation studies from the international literature, we observed also a high level of correlation between weight, fat weight, and HOMA-IR [26]. We found also that our newly defined R-ratio and Rw-ratio showed highly significant correlation with HOMA-IR, and we proposed these measures as metrics for insulin resistance [2, 3, 26]. We recognized that monitoring R-ratio and Rw-ratio may give an important tool for monitoring changes of insulin resistance; we developed CPS for this purpose. We have provided the derivation of our formulas used in CPS in the Appendix. The lists of measured and derived variables in CPS are listed in the glossary.

The essential input parameters, weight W_k and fat weight F_k, are captured by the software on MHM from a "bathroom scale" performing measurements of body composition (weight, fat weight) and hydration status (intracellular and extracellular water mass) developed by Ori Diagnostic Instruments (ODI), which is a patented apparatus for impedance spectroscopy [27, 28]. Without calorie counting and just using the required input ΔW_k, ΔF_k, and EB_k, the fat and nonfat energy balance can be estimated along with the weight-related alpha $\hat{\alpha w}_k$, the energy density parameter for weight change $\hat{\varrho_W}_k$, the weight-related Rw-ratio Rw_k, the lean mass-related alpha $\hat{\alpha}_k$, the energy density parameter for lean mass change $\hat{\varrho_L}_k$, the lean mass-related R-ratio R_k, the nonprotein respiratory quotient Rnp_k, and the fat-burning fraction χ_k as in Eqs. (1)–(19).

With additional measurement of physical activity (PAE) energy expenditure via smart watch sensors and using the measured or calculated value of the basal metabolic rate BMR_k (by either using Harris-Benedict formula or by actual measurement of BMR_k with indirect calorimetry), the total energy expenditure can be obtained as in Eq. (20).

If steady-state equilibrium in the metabolism can be assumed and the total energy expenditure is known, then it is possible to calculate food fraction φ_k, total metabolized energy intake MEI_k, fat intake FI_k, and fat oxidation FO_k in addition to $\hat{\alpha w}_k$, $\hat{\alpha}_k$, $\hat{\varrho_W}_k$, $\hat{\varrho_L}_k$, R_k, Rw_k, Rnp_k, and χ_k.

If equilibrium state is uncertain, then we would recommend additional macronutrient calorie counting on designated calibration days (maybe every 2 weeks). This could improve accuracy and would allow deeper insight into the dynamics of SVs of the metabolism.

One of the goals of this chapter is to demonstrate the feasibility of the concept of CPS for its main function which is to predict changes of insulin resistance and fat oxidation from serial measurements of weight and fat mass. Unfortunately, there is a paucity of published data with longitudinal observations and serial measurements of the measurable components of the energy metabolism including measuring markers of insulin resistance. A complete data set to study the insulin resistance and weight-fat weight relationship would require the following data: serial measurements of macronutrient energy intake (EI), total energy expenditure (TEE) and serial fat mass (F), and lean body mass (L) or weight (W) measurements. Very few trial data are published only with serial measurements of markers of insulin sensitivity or resistance. Nevertheless, we were able to identify a study suitable for our aim, which is to demonstrate the feasibility of our concept of CPS to track and predict SVs and markers of insulin resistance. Here we use published data from the study entitled "Effects of brief perturbation in energy balance on indices of glucose homeostasis in healthy lean men (EBPE) [29]."

2. Method

For all calculations I used MATLAB. To demonstrate the main functions of our CPS, we use here the published data of EBPE [29]. In this study 10 healthy men participated in two cycles of controlled 7-day periods of caloric restriction (CR) and refeeding (RF) in protocol A and overfeeding (OF) and caloric restriction (CR) in protocol B at ±60% energy requirement. Insulin resistance was assessed by HOMA-IR on the basis of measured serum insulin and glucose levels in the study participants. The mandatory input data to CPS is weight, fat weight, and daily energy balance values EB_k. The daily weights were directly scanned in from the published graphs [29]. The fat weight data points were available only at baseline and at the end of CR, RF, and OF cycles. I used MATLAB's Piecewise Cubic Hermite Interpolating Polynomial to connect these fat data points in order to have daily fat mass estimates (see **Figure 1a** and **b**). I calculated the energy balance EB_k from the difference of the metabolically utilized energy intake minus total energy expenditure.

I estimated weight-related alpha $\hat{\alpha w}_k$, energy density parameter for weight $\hat{\varrho_W}_k$, Rw-ratio Rw_k, and fat-burning fraction χ_k from ΔW_k, ΔF_k, and EB_k utilizing the methods described in Eqs. (1)–(19).

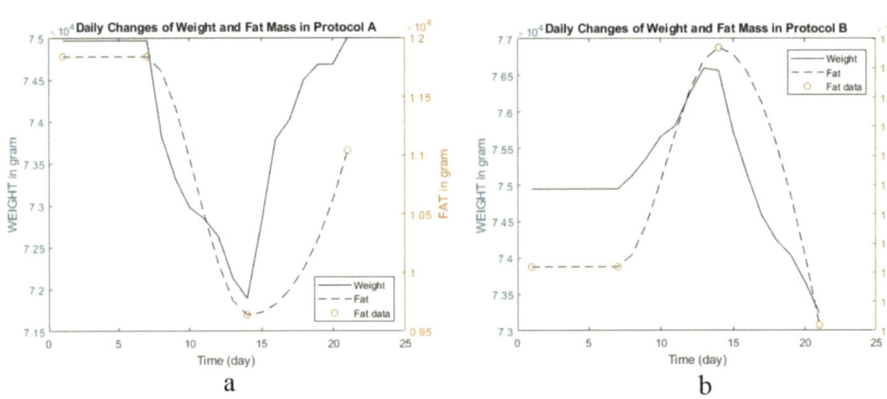

Figure 1.
(a) Daily weight and fat weight in protocol A. (b) Daily weight and fat weight in protocol B.

For calculation of correlations between HOMA-IR and weight, fat weight, R-ratio, Rw-ratio, fat-burning fraction χ_k, and nonprotein respiratory quotient Rnp_k, I used MATLAB's corrcoef function.

For demonstration purposes, I plugged the mandatory input variables ΔW_k, ΔF_k, *and* EB_k as well as the known ingested macronutrient calories CI_k, FI_k, and PI_k into SAM-HEM algorithm with Kalman filter [1–3]. As a measure of goodness of fit of the metabolic model SAM-HEM, I calculated the predicted mean value and standard deviation of the modeling error, i.e., model-predicted value minus the known trajectory of weight, fat weight, and lean mass.

3. Results

The input weight and fat weight data are shown in **Figure 1a** for Protocol A and in **Figure 1b** for Protocol B. The measured data points for fat mass are connected with MATLAB's Piecewise Cubic Hermite Interpolating Polynomial. The results of Rw-ratio Rw_k and fat-burning fractionation χ_k for Protocols A and B are in **Figure 2a** and **b**, respectively. The measured data points for HOMA-IR are connected with MATLAB's Piecewise Cubic Hermite Interpolating Polynomial.

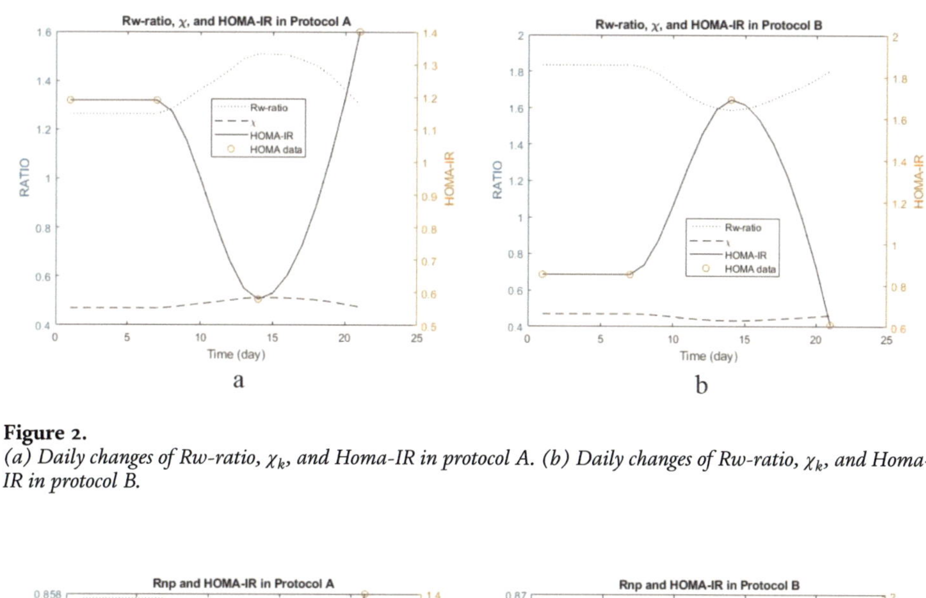

a b

Figure 2.
(a) Daily changes of Rw-ratio, χ_k, and Homa-IR in protocol A. (b) Daily changes of Rw-ratio, χ_k, and Homa-IR in protocol B.

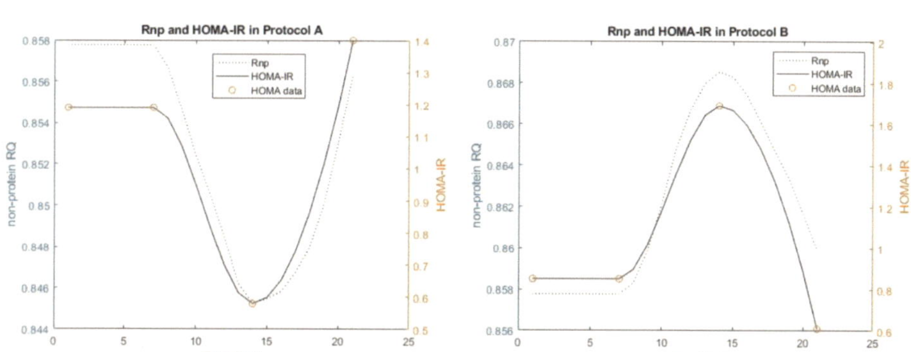

a b

Figure 3.
(a) Daily changes of Rnp and Homa-IR in protocol A. (b) Daily changes of Rnp and Homa-IR in protocol B.

In **Figure 3a** and **b**, the changes of the nonprotein respiratory quotient can be seen for Protocol A and for Protocol B. **Figure 4a** for Protocol A and **Figure 4b** for Protocol B show the results of utilized macronutrient intakes carbohydrate CI and fat FI, as well the macronutrient oxidations for carbohydrate CarbOx and fat FatOx.

The correlation coefficients between HOMA-IR and W_k, F_k, R_k, Rw_k, Rnp_k, and χ_k along with their P value are shown in **Table 1**.

The results of goodness of fit of the SAM-HEM metabolic model to the known trajectory of weight, fat weight, and lean mass are shown in **Table 2**.

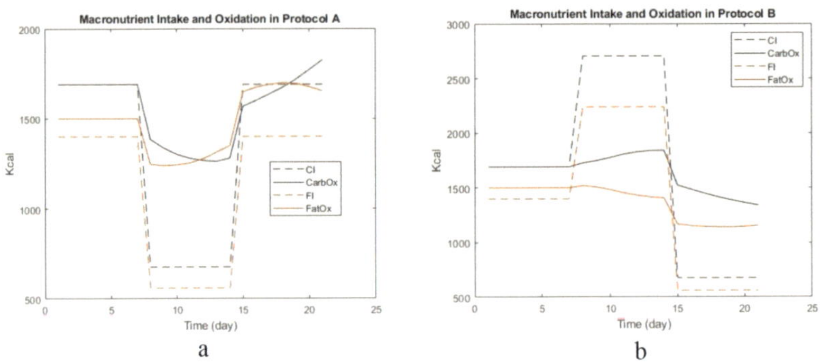

Figure 4.
(a) Daily metabolized carbohydrate and fat intake and oxidation in protocol A. (b) Daily metabolized carbohydrate and fat intake and oxidation in protocol B.

	Protocol A		Protocol B	
	HOMA-IR	**P value**	**HOMA-IR**	**P value**
W_k	0.828219114701	0.000003557891	0.6464400352912	0.00154355168
F_k	0.873415795383	0.000000235522	0.9999138255551	0.00000000000
R_k	−0.77770999896	0.000033325699	−0.971975709210	0.00000000000
Rw_k	−0.92129422123	0.000000003126	−0.967645037740	0.00000000000
Rnp_k	0.935321042397	0.000000000000	0.9529177800117	0.00000000000
χ_k	−0.9354436104	0.000000000000	−0.952802142972	0.00000000000

Table 1.
Correlation coefficients between HOMA-IR and W_k, F_k, R_k, Rw_k, Rnp_k, and χ_k.

	Protocol A		Protocol B	
	Mean deviation in grams	**Standard deviation**	**Mean deviation in grams**	**Standard deviation**
W_k	220.1045	893.8795	−289.2232	512.9418
F_k	−11.8265	122.9743	−13.3447	94.0426
L_k	21.8630	90.8594	−35.0486	40.6444

Table 2.
Goodness of fit of the SAM-HEM metabolic model to W_k, F_k, and L_k data.

4. Discussion

Insulin resistance is a pathogenic factor for type 2 diabetes. Insulin resistance has a deleterious impact on glucose and lipid metabolism, blood pressure, coagulation abnormality, inflammation, oxidative stress, and endothelial dysfunction. Population studies suggest that insulin resistance is an important target to reduce CVD risk [30]. A significant proportion of apparently healthy subjects are insulin resistant. About 30–40% of subjects are afflicted with insulin resistance in affluent countries, and the total number is over 1 billion worldwide [30]. HOMA-IR-estimated insulin resistance is associated with subsequent symptomatic CVD in the general population independent of all classic and several nontraditional risk factors [30]. The main result of EPBE [29] is that it clearly demonstrates the profound effect of energy perturbation on changes of insulin resistance. Insulin resistance remained slightly impaired at the end of Protocol A (CR followed by RF) as opposed to the end of Protocol B (OF followed by CR) where the insulin resistance created by OF was normalized by CR. As it is discussed by the authors of [29], the benefit of calorie restriction in terms of improvement of insulin sensitivity is firmly established in the medical literature in various disorders like binge eating with bulimia, weight cycling, obesity, and type II diabetes. In the EPBE study, euglycemic clamp measurements were performed parallel to the HOMA-IR. Observing these in parallel, an overarching picture emerges that the sugar and insulin dynamics are strongly connected to quantifiable dynamics of body composition and the fat metabolism as well as the carbohydrate- vs. fat-burning energy utilization.

Our feasibility demonstration for the main features of CPS is focused on assessing changes of insulin resistance. Using trial data from EBPE [29], we correlated HOMA-IR as a surrogate marker for insulin resistance with our surrogate markers such as R-ratio, Rw-ratio, 24 h nonprotein respiratory quotient, and fat-burning fraction. We found high correlation across the examined metabolic variables W_k, F_k, R_k, Rw_k, Rnp_k, and χ_k with HOMA-IR along with highly significant P value for each examined variable.

The implication is that these results show strong evidence for the feasibility for our concept to a have a noninvasive long-term monitoring tool for insulin resistance for users in their natural environment. Displaying W_k, F_k, R_k, Rw_k, Rnp_k, and χ_k on MHM and MST via our CPS can provide the needed tool to users and their providers to observe and use adaptive control strategies to improve the otherwise undetectable and invisible phenomena caused by insulin resistance and reach metabolic health.

A new method for metabolic research has been introduced here to extend the principles of indirect calorimetry to a broader application which considers serial measurements of changes of body composition and hydration status with no gas exchange measurements and is still able to estimate 24 h nonprotein respiratory quotient. For this purpose, a Lagrangian functional L was set up to establish the quantitative relationships between changes of fat mass, weight, and energy balance. Without calorie counting and just using the required input weight change ΔW_k, fat mass change ΔF_k, and energy balance EB_k, the fat and nonfat energy balance can be estimated along with important semi-stable energy parameters of the metabolism including the weight-related alpha $\hat{\alpha w}_k$, the energy density parameter for weight change $\hat{\varrho_W}_k$, the weight-related Rw-ratio Rw_k, the lean mass-related alpha $\hat{\alpha}_k$, the energy density parameter for lean mass change $\hat{\varrho_L}_k$, the lean mass-related R-ratio R_k, the nonprotein respiratory quotient Rnp_k, and the fat-burning fraction χ_k. Finding proof for the quantitative relationship between insulin resistance and Rw_k, R_k, Rnp_k, and χ_k was difficult due to lack of previous studies [24] with the needed measurements and due to non-availability of individual data of participants of potentially qualified metabolic studies. Thompson and Slezak [25] showed first that weight and fat loss are correlated well with markers of insulin resistance/ sensitivity. Kelley et al. [22] was able to show that in vivo insulin sensitivity was related to a higher in vitro capacity for fat oxidation of skeletal muscle samples. The same author found also that the strongest predictor of improved insulin sensitivity was associated with enhanced fasting rates of fat oxidation. In this context "metabolic flexibility" in the skeletal muscles is discussed in the literature [24, 31]. One definition of metabolic flexibility is the ability to switch from fat to carbohydrate oxidation during insulin-stimulated glucose disposal. Another definition of metabolic flexibility is the capacity for the organism to adept fuel oxidation to fuel availability [31]. The opposite of metabolic flexibility is metabolic inflexibility which is an important feature of insulin resistance. In the state of insulin resistance, the fuel switching is impaired, and there is an impaired capacity to upregulate muscle lipid oxidation. Metabolic inflexibility and state of insulin resistance manifest as decreased fasting rates of fat oxidation and the lack of further suppression of fat oxidation during heightened level of insulin action postprandially [32]. A defining characteristic of metabolic inflexibility is when after a fat-rich diet, an impaired drop of overnight fasting RQ (impaired fat oxidation) can be observed. Further, insulin-resistant subjects manifest less lipid oxidation during fasting condition and greater lipid oxidation during insulin-stimulated conditions relative to non-insulin-resistant subjects. The failure to augment lipid oxidation during fasting conditions likely is a key mechanism leading to lipid accumulation within skeletal muscle [32]. Supporting evidence for impaired lipolysis, diminished fat oxidation, and metabolic inflexibility was confirmed recently in obese girls with polycystic ovary syndrome and increased insulin resistance [33].

The main likely mechanism of metabolic inflexibility is that the impaired capacity to upregulate muscle lipid oxidation in the face of high lipid supply may lead to increased muscle fat accumulation and insulin resistance [31]. Many studies have shown when people are in energy balance, the 24 h food fraction φ_k, fat-burning fraction χ_k, and nonprotein respiratory quotient Rnp_k match each other [31]. With the current technology, metabolic flexibility can be studied in a metabolic chamber by measuring RQ. The testing modalities include overnight sleep study with RQ measurement or measuring RQ in response to high-carbohydrate diet or in response to high-fat diet [31]. The overnight study can show that the subject with metabolic inflexibility would burn less fat during fasting state than the individual with normal metabolism. At least 2 days of waiting is needed for seeing a clear difference in response between flexible and inflexible individuals when dietary changes are performed because adaptive mechanisms of the body prevail initially. The person with metabolic inflexibility would burn less sugar compared with a person with metabolic flexibility in response to high-carbohydrate diet. Conversely, the fat burning is better in the normal metabolism than the impaired flexibility in response to the high-fat diet. After 6–7 days, an equilibrium sets in again, and the final RQs become indistinguishable between sufferer of inflexibility and healthy, and the 24 h food fraction φ_k and fat-burning fraction χ_k settle close to the same value [31]. In summary, it is tempting to speculate that a CPS equipped with the capability to monitor nonprotein respiratory quotient Rnp_k could detect flexibility vs. inflexibility in response to dietary challenges of the user in his or her natural environment.

It is important to point out that the energy perturbation study EPBE /34/ was done in healthy men with no confounding metabolic abnormalities. Nevertheless, the correlation analysis reveals the profound connection between insulin resistance change (as measured by HOMA-IR) and energy metabolism with manifestations of substrate utilization and fat-burning capability. This becomes significant when we want to measure metabolic flexibility and create a metric for metabolic health in general. As insulin resistance (and HOMA-IR) is connected to mortality, so is metabolic inflexibility which could be now measured outside of a metabolic laboratory. In earlier publications of ours, we found evidence for close correlation already between HOMA-IR and R-ratio in a wide variety of clinical conditions including obesity, postmenopausal state, metabolic syndrome, and prediabetes /2, 3, 24/. Data from EPBE /34/ prove now that the connection between insulin resistance and R-ratio or metabolic flexibility/inflexibility exists across human physiology and pathophysiology in health or disease. Actually, EPBE /34/ helped defining the quantifiable meaning of "metabolic health," and we have now practically usable metrics for it explaining also the title of this chapter.

It is important to consider why visceral obesity and the associated increased waist circumference are a good predictor for CVD mortality [33]. The visceral fat leads to high concentration of fatty acids which contributes to impaired liver metabolism and fatty liver. The visceral adipose tissue has been shown to be loaded with macrophages which contribute to the pro-inflammatory profile of visceral obesity which would drive endothelial dysfunction and contributes to mortality. The visceral obesity-induced lipo-toxicity eventually leads to ectopic fat depositions not just in the liver but also the heart, kidney, and also skeletal muscle [34]. For management of visceral obesity, prediabetes, metabolic syndrome, and type 2 diabetes, it is important to know that physically very active persons afflicted with these conditions experience 50% reduction of CVD risk burden [33]. Further, physical activity induces a selective mobilization of visceral adipose tissue and ectopic fat even in the absence of weight loss. Consequently, our "leap ahead" innovation to unify metabolic function assessment with cardiopulmonary fitness assessment may provide an important tool to fight for less insulin resistance and higher cardiorespiratory fitness. CPS has the promise to become a comprehensive cardiometabolic function assessment tool in freely moving individuals requiring only wearing a smart watch and using a specialized stand-up scale (high accuracy bioimpedance analyzer) for serial measurement of fat mass and weight.

Increased insulin resistance states in obesity, prediabetes, metabolic syndrome, and type 2 diabetes represent a high-risk state for CVD. Restoration of impaired insulin resistance and its manifestation of impaired glucose tolerance can significantly reduce the risk of future diabetes in prediabetics and decrease the estimated CVD risk [34]. The diabetes prevention program (DPP) [35, 36] showed a clear reduction in diabetes incidence in participants assigned to the lifestyle interventions or metformin. Actually, lifestyle intervention was about twice as effective as metformin for prevention of diabetes and was the only intervention associated with regression to normal glucose regulation. Seeing the overwhelming evidence of importance of lifestyle change, we propose to utilize a CPS-like approach as outlined in introduction to help this process. CPS can be used to observe SVs such as weight, lean body mass, fat mass, R-ratio, Rw-ratio, calculated 24 h nonprotein respiratory quotient, and fat-burning fraction from serial measurements of weight, fat mass, and daily energy balance estimates EB_k. EB_k can be obtained either as per Eq. (5) with no calorie counting requirement or for enhanced accuracy with calorie counting and measurements of the physical activity energy expenditure and following Eq. (20). As a workable answer to behavioral changes mentioned in the introduction, we propose using SVs for "(A) gold standard measure" for metabolic functioning and as "(D) outcome measures for optimization" as a foreseen requisite to make breakthroughs in the fight against obesity and insulin resistance [3, 15, 16]. The predictive power of SAM-HEM can draw trajectories of SVs and allow for trend analysis and prediction and serve as "(B) ...tools allowing for planning and executing dynamic changes of behavior," as desired by behavior scientists [15, 16]. The desire for a (C) dynamic behavior change model development using self-directed behavioral change strategies can arrive with further development of CPS using control equations like the Hamilton-Jacobi-Bellman equation for dynamic optimized control [20] and with further technologies of artificial intelligence.

The main contribution of this chapter to medicine and life science is that it lays out a framework using CPS to observe and monitor long-term SVs of the metabolism including markers of insulin resistance. The CPS approach may point to new and promising directions to find workable solutions to challenges of unhealthy metabolic conditions such as insulin resistance, obesity, prediabetes, metabolic syndrome, and type 2 diabetes.

5. Conclusion

We provided important supportive evidence for feasibility for our concept of CPS for indirectly measuring and predicting the otherwise very-difficult- or impossible-to-measure slow changes of SVs and capture them for the first time noninvasively in freely moving humans in their natural environment outside of a metabolic laboratory setting. Serial fat and weight measurements and energy calculations can help unmask changes of insulin resistance in response to user's diet and exercise habits, providing tools to measure metabolic flexibility which can be used as a surrogate marker for metabolic health. Further, CPS has the potential to estimate cardiorespiratory fitness by indirectly estimating maximum oxygen uptake from measuring heart rate reserve, heart rate variability, and pulse oximetry changes with exercise. CPS is a tool to observe the two major risk factors of CVD at the same time: metabolic health and cardiorespiratory fitness, and therefore the new term cardiometabolic health is justifiable and introduced here to emphasize the two interlinked physiological functions impacting mortality significantly. CPS can enable managed and self-improvement of cardiometabolic health. CPS armed with further technologies of control engineering and artificial intelligence can unleash the potential of digital health to help manage conditions essential to primary care and to the public at large.

Acknowledgements

We would like to express our gratitude for the valuable related discussions with Professor Dr. John Buse, UNC-Chapel Hill. Further, we would like to thank Ilona Ori, JD, Ori Diagnostic Instruments, LLC, for editorial help.

Conflict of interest

The author declares that there is no conflict of interest regarding the publication of this paper. No specific funding was provided for this research. This research was performed as part of the author's employment with Ori Diagnostic Instruments, LLC. The author is the inventor of patent [27] and patent application [28], and the patent and patent application are owned by Ori Diagnostic Instruments, LLC.

Glossary

Measured variables	
F_k	fat weight
ΔF_k	fat mass change in 24 h
W_k	weight
ΔW_k	body weight change in 24 h
EB_k	daily energy balance
Derived or estimated variables	
BMR_k	basal metabolic rate
CI_k	carbohydrate calorie intake
CO_k	oxidized carbohydrate calories
ECW_k	extracellular water mass
FI_k	fat intake
FO_k	oxidized fat calories
ICW_k	intracellular water mass
L_k	lean mass
ΔL_k	lean mass change in 24 h
MEI_k	metabolically utilized energy intake
PAE_k	physical activity energy expenditure via smart watch sensors
TEE_k	total energy expenditure
R_k	R-ratio
Rw_k	Rw-ratio
Rnp_k	nonprotein respiratory quotient
α_k	first-order term coefficient of the lean body—fat logarithmic relationship Tylor series expansion
$\hat{\alpha}_k$	estimation of α_k
αw_k	first-order term coefficient of the weight—fat logarithmic relationship Tylor series expansion
$\hat{\alpha w}_k$	estimation of αw_k
$\varrho_F \approx 9.4$ Kcal/g	energy density for fat
$\varrho_L \approx 1.8$ Kcal/g	the energy density for lean mass
$\hat{\varrho}_{Lk}$	estimation of ϱ_L
ϱ_{Wk}	energy density for weight
$\hat{\varrho}_{Wk}$	estimation of ϱ_{Wk}
φ_k	fat intake fraction
χ_k	fat-burning fraction

A. Appendix

The following mathematical descriptions use elementary mathematics and a minimum set of assumptions, similar to the landmark article of [37]. These equations could be regarded as an extension of the work of [37], with my main points being that the fat-burning fraction can be calculated from serial fat and weight changes, producing the same result as 24 h indirect calorimetry. Importantly, the equations allow the clinician to determine the nonprotein respiratory quotient with serial weight and fat weight measurement, avoiding the necessity for gas exchange analysis. An important advantage of this mathematical method is that it can be used anywhere outside of a metabolic laboratory.

The R-ratio for modeling of the insulin resistance is defined in our analysis as the ratio of lean body mass change velocity ΔL_k (lean mass change in 24 h) and fat mass change velocity ΔF_k (fat mass change in 24 h) of day k as in Eq. (1).

$$R_k = \frac{\Delta L_k}{\Delta F_k}. \tag{1}$$

Likewise, Rw-ratio can be defined as the ratio of weight change velocity ΔW_k (body weight change in 24 h) and fat mass change velocity ΔF_k (fat mass change in 24 h) of day k as in Eq. (2).

$$Rw_k = \frac{\Delta W_k}{\Delta F_k}. \tag{2}$$

We proposed the Rw-ratio for modeling of the insulin resistance as it is easier to measure change of weight than lean mass [26].

The total energy balance for the day k can be expressed as in Eq. (3):

$$\varrho_{Wk} \cdot \Delta W_k + \varrho_F \cdot \Delta F_k = MEI_k - TEE_k. \tag{3}$$

The same energy balance as in (3) can be expressed also using Rw-ratio or Rw_k as in Eq. (4):

$$\left(\varrho_{Wk} \cdot Rw_k + \varrho_F\right) \cdot \Delta F_k = MEI_k - TEE_k = EB_k. \tag{4}$$

According to (3) and (4), the total energy balance (metabolically utilized energy intake MEI_k minus total energy expenditure TEE_k) is connected to changes of weight ΔW_k and body fat mass change ΔF_k at the end of day k where the energy distribution is governed by the energy density parameter for weight ϱ_{Wk} and fat ϱ_F. In the case of positive energy balance, ΔL_k, ΔW_k, and ΔF_k will have a positive sign, otherwise negative. ϱ_F is the daily energy density of the fat mass change which is estimated to be $\varrho_F \approx 9.4$ Kcal/g. Rw_k and ϱ_{Wk} need to be estimated as direct measurement is not possible. The main idea and proposition here are to estimate Rw_k from serial weight and fat weight measurement. ϱ_{Wk} is estimated here from serial measurement of weight and energy balance EB_k. Accordingly, the input to our models is going to be known measured values of daily weight W_k and fat weight F_k. The daily energy balance EB_k is indirectly measured or calculated. If no calorie counting and total energy expenditure measurements are done, then the option exists to use (5):

$$EB_k \approx (\varrho_L \cdot R_k + \varrho_F) \cdot \Delta F_k. \tag{5}$$

Here the energy density value of lean mass change ϱ_L is used, which is assumed to be around $\varrho_L \approx 1.8$ Kcal/g and is a semi-stable value [19]. Now the estimation of R_k and Rw_k is needed. Here we exploit the observation that there is a logarithmic relationship between lean mass and fat mass according to Forbes [38]:

$$L_k = \alpha_k \cdot \ln(F_k). \tag{6}$$

The same assumption can be used for weight and fat weight interrelationship:

$$W_k = \alpha w_k \cdot \ln(F_k). \tag{7}$$

Now the daily lean mass change ΔL_k can be connected to the daily fat change ΔF_k using the first-order term coefficient in the Taylor series expansion. It is noteworthy that this calculation avoids the division by zero for cases when there is no change of fat mass.

$$R_k = \frac{\Delta L_k}{\Delta F_k} \approx \frac{\alpha_k}{F_k}. \tag{8}$$

Here alpha α_k is the first-order term coefficient in the Taylor series expansion of the lean body-fat logarithmic functional relationship. For the value of $\alpha = 10.4$ is used [38] if mass is measured in kilograms. Though intuitively it is felt that this may not be the case for everybody every time, the stability assumption for α over prolonged time is made by multiple authors [19, 38, 39]. Obviously, finding the individual applicable value of α_k is desired [19].

Now, the daily weight change ΔW_k can be connected to the daily fat change ΔF_k using the first-order term coefficient in the Taylor series expansion similar to Eq. (8).

$$Rw_k = \frac{\Delta W_k}{\Delta F_k} \approx \frac{\alpha w_k}{F_k}. \tag{9}$$

Obviously, finding the individual applicable value of the semi-stable daily lean mass change-related alpha α_k, weight-related alpha αw_k, and ϱ_{Wk} is needed. For this purpose we want to take advantage of the principle of "least action" or "stationary action," which is assumed to hold true at steady state of an energy system. The same principle is widely used in Lagrangian or Hamiltonian mechanical systems. We want to extend this variational principle to the thermodynamic system of the human energy metabolism. Briefly stated, the time integral of a thermodynamic energy functional (Lagrangian functional) of the observed energy system under stationary assumption will assume a minimum value. The justification for our approach is that the first and second laws of thermodynamics (Hess's law) are fully applicable for indirect calorimetry as well as thermic energy calculations [37, 40]. The use of the principle of "least action/stationary action" will predict that the energy metabolism works with the minimum consumption of fuel and would not waste energy unnecessarily. Here we introduce our thermodynamic Lagrangian functional where the time integral is replaced by summation of energies for each day from day $k = 1$ to day $k = N$:

$$\begin{aligned} L = \sum_{k=0}^{k=N} &\left[\left(\varrho_{Wk} \cdot Rw_k + \varrho_F\right) \cdot \Delta F_k\right]^2 + \lambda\alpha w_k \cdot \left[\Delta W_k - \alpha w_k \cdot (\ln F_k - \ln F_{k-1})\right] \\ &+ \lambda\varrho_{Wk} \cdot \left[EB_k - \varrho_{Wk} \cdot \Delta W_k - \varrho_F \cdot \Delta F_k\right]. \end{aligned} \tag{10}$$

The minimum solution of L is sought for very slow changing semi-stable αw_k and ϱ_{Wk} for known ΔF_k, ΔW_k, and EB_k. This solution could be obtained with numerical methods to minimize the Lagrangian functional L. The Lagrange multipliers $\lambda\alpha w_k$ and $\lambda\varrho_{Wk}$ are non-zero variables and are part of the minimization procedure, and they multiply the constraints for conservation of mass and energy, respectively. Metabolic studies suggest that a new steady state of equilibrium ensues in 5–6 days [31] after a change of input variables occurs and equilibrium is reached. The parameters αw_k and ϱ_{Wk} can be considered stable. The Lagrangian functional L may also contain the parameter α_k in a similar fashion to αw_k if needed. Instead of using head-on numerical minimization methods to find the semi-stable parameters αw_k and ϱ_{Wk}, I prefer using the recursive least square method (RLS) of the general form $y_k = \hat{z} \cdot x_k$ where the time-dependent variables y_k and x_k are known and estimate for parameter $\hat{z}$ is sought. RLS has the advantage that the estimate of $\hat{z}_{k-1}$ at time $k-1$ can be updated at the arrival of the new measured variables y_k and x_k. This method allows us to estimate $\hat{\alpha w}_k$ when ΔW_k, ΔF_k, and F_k are available. Similarly, $\hat{\varrho_{W k}}$ can be estimated when a new set of ΔW_k, ΔF_k, and EB_k are available.

Once all parameters of the energy balance Eq. (4) are known, the nonfat energy balance and fat energy balance can be calculated as in Eqs. (11) and (12), respectively:

$$\varrho_{Wk} \cdot \Delta W_k = (1-\varphi_k) \cdot MEI_k - (1-\chi_k) \cdot TEE_k, \tag{11}$$

$$\varrho_F \cdot \Delta F_k = \varphi_k \cdot MEI_k - \chi_k \cdot TEE_k. \tag{12}$$

Here φ_k designates fat intake fraction as defined in Eq. (13), and χ_k denotes the fat-burning fraction as in Eq. (14).

$$\varphi_k = \frac{FI_k}{MEI_k}, \tag{13}$$

and

$$\chi_k = \frac{FO_k}{TEE_k}. \tag{14}$$

In Eq. (13), FI_k represents fat intake, and in Eq. (14), FO_k stands for oxidized fat calories of day k.

We made an important observation in [2, 3, 26] that the R-ratio R_k strongly and negatively correlates with HOMA-IR. Building on this observation and using Rw-ratio Rw_k, we introduce here a possible modeling of the connection between insulin resistance and substrate fractionation. At assumed steady state, the fat-burning fraction χ_k approximates food fraction φ_k according to [31], and they become quasi equal. Under this condition the nonfat and fat energy balance can be written in a simplified form as in Eqs. (15) and (16):

$$\varrho_{Wk} \cdot \Delta W_k = \frac{\varrho_F}{\varrho_{Wk} \cdot Rw_k + \varrho_F} \cdot (MEI_k - TEE_k), \tag{15}$$

$$\varrho_F \cdot \Delta F_k = \frac{\varrho_{Wk} \cdot Rw_k}{\varrho_{Wk} \cdot Rw_k + \varrho_F} \cdot (MEI_k - TEE_k). \tag{16}$$

Accordingly, the carbohydrate burning fraction $1-\chi_k$ and the fat-burning fraction χ_k can be written as in Eqs. (17) and (18):

$$1-\chi_k = \frac{\varrho_F}{\varrho_{Wk} \cdot Rw_k + \varrho_F} = \frac{CO_k}{CO_k + FO_k}, \tag{17}$$

$$\chi_k = \frac{\varrho_{Wk} \cdot Rw_k}{\varrho_{Wk} \cdot Rw_k + \varrho_F} = \frac{FO_k}{CO_k + FO_k}. \tag{18}$$

Important properties of Eqs. (15) and (16) are that they add up to the total energy balance equation as in Eq. (3). It can be seen in this pair of equations that with decreasing insulin resistance, i.e., decreasing HOMA-IR and concomitantly increasing Rw-ratio Rw_k, the fat-burning fraction χ_k increases, and the carbohydrate burning fraction $1-\chi_k$ would decrease. Similarly, with increasing insulin resistance, i.e., increasing HOMA-IR and concomitantly decreasing Rw-ratio Rw_k, the fat-burning fraction χ_k decreases, and carbohydrate burning fraction $1-\chi_k$ would increase as demonstrated in **Figure 2a** and **b**.

Further, according to Elia and Livesey [37] during nonprotein energy production, the nonprotein respiratory quotient Rnp_k can be calculated from the fat-burning fraction χ_k using stoichiometry under the assumption that mainly dioleylpalmityltriglyceride and glucose are used as fuels for oxidation as in Eq. (19) adopted from Elia [37].

$$Rnp_k = \frac{a - \chi_k \cdot a + \chi_k \cdot b \cdot c}{a - \chi_k \cdot a + \chi_k \cdot b}. \tag{19}$$

The constant values in [37] are $a = 19.502$, $b = 21.120$, and $c = 0.7097$.

All calculations from Eqs. (1)–(19) use the same assumption as Elia and Livesey [37] for their formulas, which remain in keeping and coincide with traditional indirect calorimetry calculation as introduced by Lusk [37].

The somewhat arbitrary looking choice of definitions Eqs. (17) and (18) can be justified with our experience that increasing insulin resistance would lead to more sugar burning and less fat burning. Further it allows for the calculated burning fraction χ_k in Eq. (18) to be used as an input variable to calculate the nonprotein respiratory quotient Rnp_k as in Eq. (19). The result of this choice is also that an increasing (or decreasing) burning fraction χ_k would translate into a decreasing (or increasing) nonprotein respiratory quotient Rnp_k as demonstrated in **Figure 2a** and **b** and **3a** and **b**.

We calculate the total energy expenditure as in Eq. (20):

$$TEE_k = PAE_k + BMR_k. \tag{20}$$

Author details

Zsolt Peter Ori
Ori Diagnostic Instruments, LLC, Durham, NC, USA

*Address all correspondence to: zsolt.ori56@gmail.com

References

[1] Őri Z. Parametric recursive system identification and self-adaptive modeling of the human energy metabolism for adaptive control of fat weight. Medical and Biological Engineering and Computing. 2017;**55**:(5):759-767. ISSN:0140-0118; EISSN: 1741-0444:1-9. DOI: 10.1007/s11517-016-1552-3

[2] Ori Z, Ori I. Canonical representation of the human energy metabolism of lean mass, fat mass, and insulin resistance. In: 2016 IEEE 7th Annual Ubiquitous Computing, Electronics & Mobile Communication Conference (UEMCON); IEEE; 2016. pp.1-8. ISBN: 1509014969, 9781509014965; EISBN: 1509014969, 9781509014965; DOI: 10.1109/UEMCON.2016.777786

[3] Ori Z, Ori I. Fighting weight problems and insulin resistance with the metabolic health monitor app for patients in the setting of limited access to health care in rural America. In: 2016 IEEE Global Humanitarian Technology Conference (GHTC); IEEE; 2016. pp. 547-554. ISBN: 1-5090-2433-6, 978-1-5090-2433-9; DOI: 10.1109/GHTC.2016.7857334 (IEEE Xplore All Conference Proceeding)

[4] Barquera S, Schillinger D, Aguilar-Salinas CA, Schenker M, Rodríguez LA, Hernández-Alcaraz C, et al. Collaborative research and actions on both sides of the US-Mexico border to counteract type 2 diabetes in people of Mexican origin. Globalization and Health. 2018;**14**(84):1-10. DOI: 10.1186/s12992-018-0390-5

[5] Menke A, Casagrande S, Geiss L, Cowie CC. Prevalence of and trends in diabetes among adults in the United States, 1988–2012. Journal of the American Medical Association. 2015; **314**:1021-1029

[6] Villalpando S, Shamah-Levy T, Rojas R, Aguilar-Salinas CA. Trends for type 2 diabetes and other cardiovascular risk factors in Mexico from 1993–2006. Salud Publica de Mexico. 2010;**52** (Supp. 1):S72-S79

[7] GBD 2013 Mortality and Causes of Death Collaborators. Global, regional, and national age-sex specific all-cause and cause-specific mortality for 240 causes of death, 1990–2013: A systematic analysis for the Global Burden of Disease Study 2013. Lancet. 2015;**385**:117-171

[8] Brodesser-Akner T. Losing it in the anti-dieting age: The agonies of being overweight—or running a diet company —in a culture that likes to pretend it only cares about health, not size [Internet]. The New York Times. 2017. Available from: https://nyti.ms/2uiOjYv

[9] Després J-P. Body fat distribution and risk of cardiovascular disease: An update circulation. 2012;**126**(10):1301-1313. DOI: 10.1161/CIRCULATIONAHA.111.067264

[10] Carnethon MR, De Chavez PJD, Biggs ML, Lewis CE, Pankow JS, Bertoni AG, et al. Association of weight status with mortality in adults with incident diabetes. Journal of the American Medical Association. 2012;**308**(6):581-590. DOI: 10.1001/jama.2012.9282

[11] Khan SS, Ning H, Wilkins JT, Allen N, Carnethon M, Berry JD, et al. Association of body mass index with lifetime risk of cardiovascular disease and compression of morbidity. JAMA Cardiology. 2018;**3**(4):280-287. DOI: 10.1001/jamacardio.2018.0022s

[12] Dallongeville J, Bhatt DL, Steg PH, Ravaud P, Wilson PW, Eagle KA, et al. Relation between body mass index, waist circumference, and cardiovascular

outcomes in 19,579 diabetic patients with established vascular disease: The REACH registry. European Journal of Preventive Cardiology. 2012;**19**:241-249

[13] Godsland IF, Lecamwasam K, Johnston DG. A systematic evaluation of the insulin resistance syndrome as an independent risk factor for cardiovascular disease mortality and derivation of a clinical index. Metabolism. 2011;**60**(10):1442-1448. DOI: 10.1016/j.metabol.2011.02.012. [Epub 2011 Apr 2]

[14] Arena R, Guazzi M, Lianov L, Whitsel L, Berra K, Lavie CJ, et al. Healthy lifestyle interventions to combat noncommunicable disease—A novel nonhierarchical connectivity model for key stakeholders: A policy statement from the American Heart Association, European Society of Cardiology, European Association for Cardiovascular Prevention and Rehabilitation, and American College of Preventive Medicine. Mayo Clinic Proceedings. 2015;**90**(8):1082-1103

[15] Spruijt-Metz D et al. Building new computational models to support health behavior change and maintenance: New opportunities in behavioral research. Translational Behavioral Medicine. 2015;**5**(3):335-346. DOI: 10.1007/s13142-015-0324-1

[16] Riley WT. Health behavior models in the age of mobile interventions: Are our theories up to the task? Translational Behavioral Medicine. 2011;**1**(1):53-71. DOI: 10.1007/s13142-011-0021-7

[17] Hall KD. Computational model of in vivo human energy metabolism during semistarvation and refeeding. American Journal of Physiology-Endocrinology and Metabolism. 2006; **291**(1):E23-E37

[18] Hall KD. Predicting metabolic adaptation, body weight change, and energy intake in humans. American Journal of Physiology-Endocrinology and Metabolism. 2010;**298**(3): E449-E466

[19] Hall KD. Mechanisms of metabolic fuel selections. IEEE Engineering in Medicine and Biology Magazine. 2010; **28**(1):36-41

[20] Kirk DE. Optimal Control Theory. An Introduction. Mineola, New York: Dover Publications, Inc.; ISBN 0-486-43484-2

[21] Grewal MS, Andrews AP. Kalman Filtering Theory and Practice Using MATLAB. 3rd ed. New Jersey: John Wiley & Sons; 2008

[22] Kelley DE, Goodpaster B, Wing RR, Simoneau J-A. Skeletal muscle fatty acid metabolism in association with insulin resistance, obesity, and weight loss. American Journal of Physiology-Endocrinology and Metabolism. 1999; **277**(40):E1130-E1141

[23] Goldsmith R, Joanisse DR, Gallagher D, Pavlovich K, Shamoon E, Leibel RL, et al. Effects of experimental weight perturbation on skeletal muscle work efficiency, fuel utilization, and biochemistry in human subjects. American Journal of Physiology. Regulatory, Integrative and Comparative Physiology. 2010;**298**: R79-R88

[24] Müller MJ, Lagerpusch M, Enderle J, Schautz B, Heller M, Bosy-Westphal A. Beyond the body mass index: Tracking body composition in the pathogenesis of obesity and the metabolic syndrome. Obesity Reviews. 2012;**13**(2):6-13; ISSN: 1467-7881, EISSN: 1467-789X. DOI: 10.1111/j.1467-789X.2012.01033.x

[25] Thompson WG, Slezak JM. Correlations between measures of insulin sensitivity and weight loss. Diabetes Research and Clinical Practice. 2006;**74**(2):129-134

[26] Ori Z. The predictability of insulin resistance and fat oxidation changes from serial measurements of weight and fat mass. In: Annual Scientific Meeting in Sarasota, Florida of the Hungarian Medical Association of America. October 28-November 2, 2018. Vol. 26. 2018. Arch. Hun. Med. Assoc. Am., 2018;**26**(3):92. ISSN 1070-0773

[27] Ori Z. An apparatus and method for the analysis of the change of body composition and hydration status and for dynamic indirect individualized measurement of components of the human energy metabolism. U.S. Patent No.: US 9,949,663 B1 2018

[28] Ori Z. Systems and methods for high frequency impedance spectroscopy detection of daily changes of dielectric properties of the human body to measure body composition and hydration status. U.S. Patent Application Publication. No: US 2017/0340239 A1 2017

[29] Lagerpusch M, Bosy-Westphal A, Kehden B, Peters A, Mueller MJ. Effects of brief perturbations in energy balance on indices of glucose homeostasis in healthy lean men. International Journal of Obesity. 2012;**36**(8):1094-1101

[30] Bonora E, Kiechl S, Willeit J, Oberhollenzer F, Egger G, Meigs JB, et al. Insulin resistance as estimated by homeostasis model assessment predicts incident symptomatic cardiovascular disease in caucasian subjects from the general population: The Bruneck study. Diabetes Care. 2007;**30**(2):318-324. DOI: 10.2337/dc06-0919

[31] Galgani JE, Moro C, Ravussin E. Metabolic flexibility and insulin resistance. American Journal of Physiology—Endocrinology and Metabolism. 2008;**295**(5):1009-1017; ISSN: 0193-1849, EISSN: 1522-1555. DOI: 10.1152/ajpendo.90558.2008

[32] Kelley DE, Mandarino LJ. Fuel selection in human skeletal muscle in insulin resistance. A Reexamination. Diabetes. 2000;**49**(5):677-683

[33] Kim JY, Tfayli H, Michaliszyn SF, Arslanian S. Impaired lipolysis, diminished fat oxidation, and metabolic inflexibility in obese girls with polycystic ovary syndrome. Journal of Clinical Endocrinology & Metabolism. 2018;**103**(2):546-554. DOI: 10.1210/jc.2017-01958

[34] Myers J, McAuley P, Lavie CJ, Despres JP, Arena R, Kokkinos P. Physical activity and cardiorespiratory fitness as major markers of cardiovascular risk: Their independent and interwoven importance to health status. Progress in Cardiovascular Diseases. 2015;**57**(4):306-314. DOI: 10.1016/j.pcad.2014.09.011 (Epub Sep 28, 2014)

[35] Perreault L, Temprosa M, Mather KJ, Horton E, Kitabchi A, Larkin M, et al. Regression from prediabetes to normal glucose regulation is associated with reduction in cardiovascular risk: Results from the diabetes prevention program outcomes study. Diabetes Care. 2014;**37**(9):2622-2631. DOI: 10.2337/dc14-0656 (Epub Jun 26, 2014)

[36] Knowler WC, Barrett-Connor E, Fowler SE, Hamman RF, Lachin JM, Walker EA, et al. Reduction in the incidence of type 2 diabetes with lifestyle intervention or metformin. New England Journal of Medicine. 2002;**346**(6):393-403. DOI: 10.1056/NEJMoa012512

[37] Elia M, Livesey G. Theory and validity of indirect calorimetry during net lipid synthesis. American Journal of Clinical Nutrition. 1988;**47**(4):591-607; ISSN: 0002-9165, EISSN:1938-3207. DOI: 10.1093/ajcn/47.4.591

[38] Forbes GB. Lean body mass-body fat interrelationships in humans. Nutrition Reviews. 1987;**45**(8):225-231

[39] Guo J, Hall KD. Estimating the continuous-time dynamics of energy

and fat metabolism in mice. PLoS Computational Biology. 2009;**5**(9):1-7: e1000511. DOI: 10.1371/journal.pcbi.1000511

[40] Simonson DC, DeFronzo RA. Indirect calorimetry: Methodological and interpretative problems. American Journal of Physiology—Endocrinology and Metabolism. 1990;**258**(3); ISSN: 0193-1849, 0002-9513, EISSN: 1522-1555, 2163-5773. DOI: 10.1152/ajpendo.1990.258.3.E399

Chapter 8

Health Information Technologies in Diabetes Management

Yilin Yoshida and Eduardo J. Simoes

Abstract

About 1 in 11 adults worldwide now have diabetes mellitus, 90% of whom have type 2 diabetes (T2D). Successful glycemic control helps to prevent and reduce complications of T2D, including cardiovascular disease, kidney disease, blindness, neuropathy, and limb amputation, and reduce death related to the disease. However, maintaining optimal glycemic control requires ongoing monitoring and treatment, which can be costly and challenging. To improve diabetes management, the development of innovative self-care strategies is warranted. Advances in health information technologies (HITs) have introduced approaches that support effective and affordable health-care delivery and patient education. Technologies in mobile, computer, e-mail, and Internet approaches have shown evidence in enhancing chronic disease management, suggesting great potential for diabetes management technologies. In this chapter, we provided an overview of the HITs in use for T2D management. We synthesized the latest findings on HITs' effect in reducing HbA1c and managing complications, cardiovascular conditions, in particular. Further, we discussed limitations in the current research in this area and implications for future research. Last, we presented challenges of applying HITs in T2D management in the real-world context and suggested steps to move forward.

Keywords: health information technologies, type 2 diabetes mellitus, glycemic control, HbA1c

1. Introduction

Diabetes is the fastest growing chronic condition worldwide. The prevalence of people with type 2 diabetes (T2D) is growing in each country [1]. Diabetes is also the seventh leading cause of deaths in the world. Around 1.6 million people died due to diabetes in 2016 [1]. Higher blood glucose levels also caused an additional 2.2 million deaths, by increasing the risks of cardiovascular and other complications such as kidney disease, blindness, neuropathy, and limb amputation [2–4]. Successful glycemic control can prevent and reduce these complications. However, to maintain optimal glycemic control requires ongoing monitoring and treatment, which can be costly and challenging [5]. Advances in health information technologies (HITs) have introduced approaches that support effective and affordable health-care delivery and education. Technologies in mobile, computer, e-mail, and Internet approaches have shown evidence in enhancing chronic disease management including diabetes management, via supporting provider decision-making (through electronic risk assessment, alerts, guidelines, formularies, and prescribing) and facilitating patient self-management (through risk communication, Web portals, telemedicine, e-mailing, and secure messaging) [6–8]. In this chapter, we summarized the current findings on HITs in managing T2D, especially on glycemic control and CVD risks management. In addition, we discussed limitations in the current research in this area and implications for future research. Further, we presented challenges of applying HITs in T2D management in the real-world context and suggested steps to move forward.

2. The potential of HITs in chronic disease management

HITs include a broad range of technologies, electronic tools, applications, or systems that provide patient care, information, recommendations, or services for promotion of health and health care [9]. The advantages of using HITs in health care have been well documented [10–13]. They have the potential to empower patients and support a transition from a role in which the patient is the passive recipient of care services to an active role in which the patient is informed, has choices, and is involved in the decision-making process [10]. They are also designed to promote communication and relationships between clinicians and patients and overcome geographical barriers and logistical inconvenience when seeking health-care services [11]. In the realm of chronic disease management, a variety of technologies have shown their positive effects. For examples, electronic health record system provides reminders at the point of care for providers to identify high-priority clinical areas for patients with complex chronic illness [14]; telemonitoring system provides asthma patients with continuous individualized help in the daily routine of asthma self-care [12]; Web-based applications increase knowledge, problem-solving skills, and social support via an interactive system for patients with cancers [13]; mobile technology devices such as personal digital assistants (PDAs) and cellular phones enable additional resources to care and change the location of care; and mobile phone short message service (SMS) were able to remind patients of scheduled visits, deliver test results, and monitor side effects of treatment [15–17]. The HIT-enabled self-care keeps evolving and attempts to address more challenging health-care issues, such as diabetes management where patients need comprehensive information and ongoing guidance as they work to develop a diverse knowledge and skills.

3. HITs in glycemic control among patients with T2D

A growing research attention has been given to evaluate HITs' impact on diabetes management, including the primary management goal, glycemic status, and major complications such as cardiovascular conditions. Previous reviews on this subject suggested that HITs have the potential to improve these disease outcomes [18–23]. However, effect size is specific to the main outcome; glycated hemoglobin (HbA1c) varied between studies with reported mean difference ranging from −0.20 to −0.57% [19–23]. **Table 1** presented the synthesized findings from the latest systematic reviews. Heitkemper et al. searched randomized control trials (RCTs) that studied the effect of HITs on HbA1c among medically underserved patients [21]. In this meta-analysis of 10 eligible trials, HITs were associated with significant HbA1c reduction at 6 months (pooled standardized difference in mean: −0.36, 95% CI −0.53, −0.19) with diminishing but still significant effect at 12 months (pooled standardized difference in mean: −0.27, 95% CI −0.49, −0.04). The authors also performed analyses by HIT type including computer software without Internet

Author, year	Objective and intervention(s) under review	Inclusion criteria	Sample	HbA1c reduction (absolute difference in means)	HbA1c reduction (standardized difference in means and Hedges' g)	CVD risk factor assessment	Intervention period	HIT subgroup analysis	Major limitations
Yoshida et al., 2018 [33]	Evaluating of effect of HITs on T2D glycemic control in general T2D patients, including mobile phone-based HITs, Web-based HITs, short message/ text, and other HITs	RCTs conducted from 1946 to December 2017	34 RCTs (40 estimation points); 3983 participants with T2D	−0.65% (95% CI −0.99, −0.64%)	Standard mean difference: −0.57 (95% CI −0.71, −0.43); Hedges' g: −0.56 (95% CI −0.70, −0.43)	A separate analysis focusing on CVD risk factors is upcoming	2–12 months	Mobile phone-based approaches [Hedges' g = −0.66 (95% CI −0.88, −0.45)]; SMS/text [Hedges' g = −0.63 (95% CI −1.07, −0.19)]; Web-based [Hedges' g = −0.48 (95% CI −0.65, −0.30)]	Did not provide analysis at different time points
Heitkemper et al., 2017 [21]	Evaluating of effect of HIT self-management interventions on glycemic control in medically underserved adults with diabetes, including computer software without Internet, cellular/ automated telephone, Internet-based HITs, and telemedicine/ telehealth	RCTs conducted from 2000 to 2015	10 RCTs; 3257 medically underserved adults with diabetes	Not reported	Standard mean difference: −0.36, 95% CI −0.53, −0.19 at 6 months and −0.27, 95% CI −0.49, −0.04 at 12 months	No	Up to 12 months	Internet-based HITs (standard mean difference = −0.50, 95% CI −0.69, −0.32 at 6 months and −0.87, 95% CI −1.58, −0.21 at 12 months); cellular/automated telephone HITs (standard mean difference = −0.26, 95% CI −0.49, −0.03 at 6 months and not significant at 12 months); telehealth (standard mean difference = −0.37, 95% CI −0.68, −0.06 at 6 months and not significant at 12 months)	External validity issue (only focused on a specific patient group); mixed participants with type 1 and 2 diabetes

Author, year	Objective and intervention(s) under review	Inclusion criteria	Sample	HbA1c reduction (absolute difference in means)	HbA1c reduction (standardized difference in means and Hedges' g)	CVD risk factor assessment	Intervention period	HIT subgroup analysis	Major limitations
Tao et al., 2017 [18]	Evacuating of effect of consumer-oriented HITs in diabetes management	RCTs conducted up until July 2016	18 RCTs; participants in trials ranged from 14 to 1382	Not reported	Standard mean difference: −0.31, 95% CI −0.38, −0.23; glycemic control was significant at intervention duration of 3, 6, 8, 9, 12, 15, 30, and 60 months	No	Up to 60 months	Not reported	Lumped all types of HITs into analysis; mixed participants with type 1 and 2 diabetes
Faruque et al., 2017 [20]	Evaluating of effect of telemedicine on glycemic control, including broad forms of electronic forms communication.	RCTs conducted from 1946 to November 2015	111 RCTs; 23,648 participants with diabetes	−0.57% (95% CI −0.74, −0.40%) at ≥3 months; −0.28% (95% −0.37, −0.20%) at 4–12 months; −0.26% (95% −0.46, −0.06%) at >12 months	Not reported	No	3–68 months	The effect was the greatest in trials where providers used Web portals or text messaging to communicate with patients [mean difference: −0.35% (95% −0.56, −0.14) and −0.28% (95% CI −0.52, −0.14)] at 4–12 months	Mixed participants with type 1 and 2 diabetes
Alharbi et al., 2016 [19]	Evaluating of effect of HITs in glycemic control in T2D patients. HITs included Web-based approaches, telephone-based system, mobile phone-based system, and telemedicine	RCTs conducted up until July 2016	32 RCTs; 40,454 participants with T2D	−0.33%, (95% CI −0.40, −0.26)	Not reported	No	3–36 months	Electronic self-management systems [mean difference: −0.50% (95% CI −0.67, −0.43%)]; EHR [mean difference: −0.33% (95% CI −0.40, −0.26%)]; electronic decision support system [mean difference: −0.15% (95% CI −0.34, −0.16%)]; diabetes registry [mean difference: −0.05% (95% CI −0.15, −0.19%)]	Did not provide analysis at different time points

Author, year	Objective and intervention(s) under review	Inclusion criteria	Sample	HbA1c reduction (absolute difference in means)	HbA1c reduction (standardized difference in means and Hedges' g)	CVD risk factor assessment	Intervention period	HIT subgroup analysis	Major limitations
Pal et al., 2014 [24]	Evaluating computer-based interventions in self-management in T2D patients. Intervention delivered via clinics, the Internet, and mobile phone	RCTs conducted up until November 2011	16 RCTs; 3578 participants with T2D	−0.2% (95% CI −0.4, −0.1%)	Not reported	Yes. Did not find improvement of blood pressure, lipids, or weight due to interventions	8 weeks to 12 months	Mobile phone intervention (mean difference: −0.5%, 95% CI −0.3, −0.7)	Did not provide analysis at different time points
Marcolino et al., 2013 [22]	Evaluating of effect of telemedicine on diabetes care	RCTs conducted up until April 2012	13 RCTs; 4207 participants with diabetes	−0.44% (95% CI −0.61, −0.26%)	Not reported	Yes. Only found telemedicine was associated with reduction in LDL (−6.6 mg/dL, 95% CI −8.3, −4.9 mg/dL)	6–18 months	Not reported	Mixed participants with type 1 and 2 diabetes; did not provide analysis at different time points
Liang et al., 2010 [23]	Evaluating of effect of mobile phone intervention for diabetes on glycemic control	RCTs conducted from January 2010 to February 2010	22 trials including 11 RCTs and 11 non-RCTs; 1657 participants with diabetes	−0.5% (95% CI −0.3, −0.7%)	Not reported	No	3–12 months	Not reported	Lumped nonrandomized and randomized trials together into evaluation

Table 1.
Synthesized findings of effect of HITs on HbA1c and cardiovascular risk factors among diabetes patients.

(n = 2), cellular/automated telephone (n = 4), Internet-based (n = 4), and telemedicine/telehealth (n = 3). The Internet-based interventions demonstrated the greatest reduction in HbA1c at both 6 months (pooled standardized difference in mean: −0.50, 95% CI −0.69, −0.32) and 12 months (pooled standardized difference in mean: −0.87, 95% CI −1.58, −0.21). Cellular and automated telephone interventions showed the smallest reduction. In Tao and colleagues' systematic review on consumer-centered HITs, they identified a significant pooled reduction of −0.31 (95% CI −0.38, −0.23) in HbA1c from 18 RCTs [18]. Similarly, Alharbi et al. also found HITs were associated with a statistically significant reduction in HbA1c levels (mean difference: −0.33%, 95% CI −0.40, −0.26%) [19]. In addition, Alharbi and colleagues found studies focusing on electronic self-management systems demonstrated the greatest reduction in HbA1c (−0.50%), followed by those with electronic medical records (−0.17%), an electronic decision support system (−0.15%), and a diabetes registry (−0.05%) [19]. Faruque et al. identified 11 RCTs with specific focus on effect of telemedicine [20]. Telemedicine refers to the use of telecommunications to deliver health services, expertise, and information on glycemic control [20]. In this study, the authors demonstrated a significant reductions in HbA1c all three follow-up periods (mean difference at ≤3 months: −0.57%, 95% CI −0.74, −0.40%, at 4–12 months: −0.28%, 95% CI −0.37, −0.20%, and at >12 months: −0.26%, 95% CI −0.46, −0.06%). In another meta-analysis that specially focused on telemedicine, Marcolino and colleagues found telemedicine was associated with a statistically significant and clinically relevant decline in HbA1c level compared to control (mean difference = −0.44%, 95% CI −0.61, −0.26%) [22]. Pal et al. examined the effect of computer-based intervention in self-management in adults with T2D. The authors found modest effect associated with the interventions (mean difference: −0.2%, 95% CI −0.4, −0.1%) [24]. Liang et al. assessed the effect of mobile phone intervention on glycemic control in diabetes self-management and found a significant common reduction of HbA1c (mean difference: −0.5%, 95% CI −0.3, −0.7%) among 22 trials over a median follow-up of 6 months [23].

Many of review studies including those mentioned above have shed light on the effect of HITs in glycemic control. However, these studies often included limited number of trials [21], lack of adherence to standard quantitative methods [25], inadequate attention to heterogeneity across studies [26], lumped nonrandomized and randomized trials together into evaluation [19, 23, 25, 27–29], mixed participants with type 1 or type 2 diabetes into analysis [18, 22, 25, 27–29], or restricted searching criteria to a particular patient population or a specific type of HIT [27, 30–32]. To address these limitations and to verify if and how much HITs impact glycemic control, Yoshida and colleagues recently conducted a meta-analysis to examine the most current state of evidence from RCTs concerning the effect of HITs on HbA1c reduction among patients with T2D [33]. From an analysis of 34 eligible studies (40 estimates) identified from multiple databases from January 1946 to December 2017, the study reported that introduction of HITs to standard diabetes treatment resulted in a statistically reduced HbA1c. The absolute mean difference in HbA1c pre- and postintervention between intervention and control group was −0.65% (95% CI −0.99, −0.64%). The pooled reduction (standardized difference in means) of HbA1c was −0.57 (95% CI −0.71, −0.43) (**Figure 1**). In addition, Yoshida et al. also found the reduction was significant across each of the four types of HIT interventions (i.e., mobile phone-based, Web-based technologies, SMS/text, or others) under review, with mobile phone-based approaches generating the largest effects [pooled reduction was −0.67 (95% CI −0.90, −0.45)] followed by SMS/text [−0.64 (95% CI −1.09, −0.19)], and Web-based [−0.48 (95% CI −0.65, −0.30)] [33].

DOI: http://dx.doi.org/10.5772/intechopen.83693

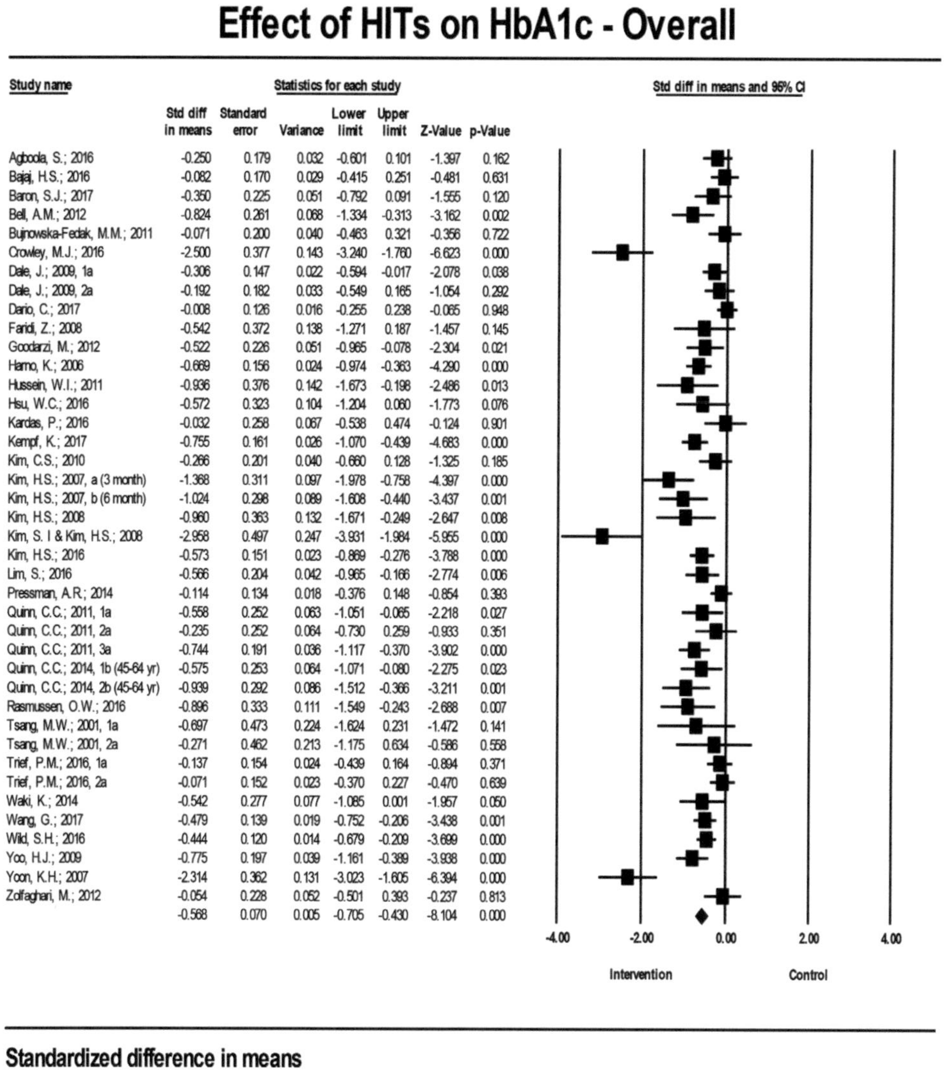

Effect of HITs on HbA1c - Overall

Study name	Std diff in means	Standard error	Variance	Lower limit	Upper limit	Z-Value	p-Value
Agboola, S.; 2016	-0.250	0.179	0.032	-0.601	0.101	-1.397	0.162
Bajaj, H.S.; 2016	-0.082	0.170	0.029	-0.415	0.251	-0.481	0.631
Baron, S.J.; 2017	-0.350	0.225	0.051	-0.792	0.091	-1.555	0.120
Bell, A.M.; 2012	-0.824	0.261	0.068	-1.334	-0.313	-3.162	0.002
Bujnowska-Fedak, M.M.; 2011	-0.071	0.200	0.040	-0.463	0.321	-0.356	0.722
Crowley, M.J.; 2016	-2.500	0.377	0.143	-3.240	-1.760	-6.623	0.000
Dale, J.; 2009, 1a	-0.306	0.147	0.022	-0.594	-0.017	-2.078	0.038
Dale, J.; 2009, 2a	-0.192	0.182	0.033	-0.549	0.165	-1.054	0.292
Dario, C.; 2017	-0.008	0.126	0.016	-0.255	0.238	-0.065	0.948
Faridi, Z.; 2008	-0.542	0.372	0.138	-1.271	0.187	-1.457	0.145
Goodarzi, M.; 2012	-0.522	0.226	0.051	-0.965	-0.078	-2.304	0.021
Harno, K.; 2006	-0.669	0.156	0.024	-0.974	-0.363	-4.290	0.000
Hussein, W.I.; 2011	-0.936	0.376	0.142	-1.673	-0.198	-2.486	0.013
Hsu, W.C.; 2016	-0.572	0.323	0.104	-1.204	0.060	-1.773	0.076
Kardas, P.; 2016	-0.032	0.258	0.067	-0.538	0.474	-0.124	0.901
Kempf, K.; 2017	-0.755	0.161	0.026	-1.070	-0.439	-4.683	0.000
Kim, C.S.; 2010	-0.266	0.201	0.040	-0.660	0.128	-1.325	0.185
Kim, H.S.; 2007, a (3 month)	-1.368	0.311	0.097	-1.978	-0.758	-4.397	0.000
Kim, H.S.; 2007, b (6 month)	-1.024	0.298	0.089	-1.608	-0.440	-3.437	0.001
Kim, H.S.; 2008	-0.960	0.363	0.132	-1.671	-0.249	-2.647	0.008
Kim, S. I & Kim, H.S.; 2008	-2.958	0.497	0.247	-3.931	-1.984	-5.955	0.000
Kim, H.S.; 2016	-0.573	0.151	0.023	-0.869	-0.276	-3.788	0.000
Lim, S.; 2016	-0.566	0.204	0.042	-0.965	-0.166	-2.774	0.006
Pressman, A.R.; 2014	-0.114	0.134	0.018	-0.376	0.148	-0.854	0.393
Quinn, C.C.; 2011, 1a	-0.558	0.252	0.063	-1.051	-0.065	-2.218	0.027
Quinn, C.C.; 2011, 2a	-0.235	0.252	0.064	-0.730	0.259	-0.933	0.351
Quinn, C.C.; 2011, 3a	-0.744	0.191	0.036	-1.117	-0.370	-3.902	0.000
Quinn, C.C.; 2014, 1b (45-64 yr)	-0.575	0.253	0.064	-1.071	-0.080	-2.275	0.023
Quinn, C.C.; 2014, 2b (45-64 yr)	-0.939	0.292	0.086	-1.512	-0.366	-3.211	0.001
Rasmussen, O.W.; 2016	-0.896	0.333	0.111	-1.549	-0.243	-2.688	0.007
Tsang, M.W.; 2001, 1a	-0.697	0.473	0.224	-1.624	0.231	-1.472	0.141
Tsang, M.W.; 2001, 2a	-0.271	0.462	0.213	-1.175	0.634	-0.586	0.558
Trief, P.M.; 2016, 1a	-0.137	0.154	0.024	-0.439	0.164	-0.894	0.371
Trief, P.M.; 2016, 2a	-0.071	0.152	0.023	-0.370	0.227	-0.470	0.639
Waki, K.; 2014	-0.542	0.277	0.077	-1.085	0.001	-1.957	0.050
Wang, G.; 2017	-0.479	0.139	0.019	-0.752	-0.206	-3.438	0.001
Wild, S.H.; 2016	-0.444	0.120	0.014	-0.679	-0.209	-3.699	0.000
Yoo, H.J.; 2009	-0.775	0.197	0.039	-1.161	-0.389	-3.938	0.000
Yoon, K.H.; 2007	-2.314	0.362	0.131	-3.023	-1.605	-6.394	0.000
Zolfaghari, M.; 2012	-0.054	0.228	0.052	-0.501	0.393	-0.237	0.813
	-0.568	0.070	0.005	-0.705	-0.430	-8.104	0.000

Standardized difference in means

Figure 1.
Pooled reduction of HbA1c due to HITs. Adopted from the study of Yoshida et al [33].

HITs also have significant clinical impact in reducing HbA1c among patients with T2D. It is reported that every 1% decrease in HbA1c over a 10-year period is associated with a risk reduction of 21% for diabetes-related death and 37% of microvascular complications [34]. This reduction results from HIT interventions may be bigger than effects of many targeted pharmacological therapies. Oral antidiabetic agents reduced HbA1c levels of 0.5–1.25%, with thiazolidinedione and sulfonylureas showing the best reduction (1–1.25%) [35]. Biguanide reduced HbA1c by 1.0–2.0%; dipeptidyl peptidase 4 (DPP-IV) inhibitor, 0.5–0.8%; GLP-1 agonists, 0.5–1.5%; and TZD, 0.5–1.4% [36]. It is questionable that the effects on HbA1c yielded from the HIT trials were a mixed product of both HITs and standard diabetes care including medication adherence and lifestyle modifications. This concern was addressed in the systematic review of Yoshida et al. [33]. The authors conducted a subset analysis of 18 studies that exclusively compared the outcome between a combined HITs and standard care intervention group vs. standard care control group. The effect size estimated from this analysis was −0.63 (Hedges' g: −0.63 95% CI −0.84, −0.42), which is attributable to HIT tools in addition to the usual care [33]. This result suggests that HITs are the key to the effectiveness rather than tools or components of these trials. Additionally, pharmacotherapies often use motivated patients' sample and they cannot generate their full effects without patients' adherence to treatment and persistence in usage [33]. In this sense, HITs may add additional value in the effectiveness by addressing challenges in adherence of a pharmacological therapy or of behavioral interventions.

4. HITs in managing cardiovascular risks among patients with T2D

T2D is commonly accompanied by cardiovascular complications. Adults with diabetes have a 77–87% prevalence of hypertension, a 74–81% prevalence of elevated low-density lipoprotein cholesterol (LDL), and a 62–67% prevalence of obesity [37]. Cardiovascular disease (CVD) is recognized as the most frequent cause of morbidity and mortality in patients with diabetes, causing up to 70% of all deaths in this patient group [2]. Type 2 diabetes (T2D) confers an approximate twofold elevation of CVD risk, equivalent to that of a previous myocardial infarction [3, 38]. In light of CVD burden in those with diabetes, the management of modifiable CVD risk factors, including hypertension, dyslipidemia, and obesity, is critical to minimizing the risk of macrovascular complications as well as death of diabetes. Yet, the implementation of preventive strategies to CVD among individuals with T2D is often not adequate [39–41] and less than half of patients who visit their care provider meet recommended levels for blood pressure (BP) and lipids [42]. Innovative approaches such as HITs are needed to facilitate CVD risk factor management among patients with T2D.

In the context of cardiovascular care among general populations, HITs were documented to offer numerous benefits and have been associated with improvements in the measurement and monitoring of heart health, including risk factors such as BP, arrhythmia, cholesterol, and weight, as well as the implementation of guideline-based decision support for providers [43]. However, CVD outcomes are usually secondary and less described compared to glycemic status in T2D management trials [26, 44]. Furthermore, many review studies examining HITs' effect in diabetes management often overlooked CVD outcomes [26, 44] or include insufficient sample size or limited CVD parameters for analysis [22, 24]. In the study by Marcolino et al., only 13 studies were included in the final analysis, within which 8 studies assessed the effect on SBP, 7 on DBP, and 5 on LDL [22]. No effects of telecommunication and information technologies were seen on SBP and DBP. They did, however, find a statistically significant reduction on LDL (−6.6 mg/dL, 95% CI −8.3, −4.9 mg/dL) associated with the technologies evaluated. They were not able to perform analysis on weight outcome, because only two studies assessed the effect of HITs on weight and both studies demonstrated a nonsignificant reduction on weight. In the systematic review by Pal et al., among 11 RCTs included in their final analysis, 5 studies looked into changes in BP (only 1 showed improvement in BP), 7 reported changes in BMI or weight (5 were combined in a meta-analysis), and 10 measured serum lipids (7 were combined in a meta-analysis) [24]. The overall pooled effect did not reach statistical significance for all of these outcomes [24].

5. Research limitations and implications

The current research on the effect of HITs in diabetes management has several limitations. First of all, the published trials often do not provide protocols for studies [45]. There is also lack of information on the theoretical bases of the interventions, and whether the HIT interventions are accompanied by other pharmaceutical or lifestyle therapies in their publications. As these HIT interventions are main therapeutic agents, it would be beneficial to explicitly prescribe interventions for trials and state the active components (behavior-change techniques), dose (frequency and intensity of interactions), route (mode of delivery), and duration of treatment [45]. There is also a need to clarify other ingredients in the intervention such as medication, standard care from health professionals, so that the major role of the HITs to the effectiveness of the interventions can be estimated, separating the effects from usual care and treatment [33].

Additionally, intervention periods in published trials are short (most trials under 1 year) [33] and few systematic reviews provided effect estimation by length of follow-up. Studies by Tao et al. and Heitkemper et al. showed that HITs' effect on glycemic control was diminishing as the interventions proceeded [18, 21]. It is not clear whether intervention effect and compliance with the HIT interventions would sustain in the long term. Misuse or nonuse of technological support is a common problem in disease management, which greatly affects patient's outcomes. There is also lack of focus on cardiovascular health assessments in HIT interventions for diabetes management. We only found two systematic reviews that discussed CVD outcomes in addition to glycemic control. Because very few trials included cardiovascular risk factor evaluations, the synthesized findings were modest (**Table 1**). As we discussed earlier, because CVD causes major morbidity and mortality among T2D patients, designing and evaluating HITs for diabetes management should include cardiovascular health indicators. Further, many review studies only reported standardized difference in means [18, 21], which may be less intuitive to patients who care the absolute changes (i.e., mean difference) in outcomes (e.g., HbA1c) due to an intervention. Moreover, it remains unclear whether there are harms associated with the intervention. It has been reported that people may suffer from negative consequences of excessive self-monitoring by finding it uncomfortable, intrusive, and unpleasant [46, 47]. Studies found patients with diabetes who self-monitor their own blood glucose concentration did not benefit from increased glycemic control but rather found their disease more intrusive [48]. The interaction between a HIT device and a patient can be complex, and further studies need to consider these in more detail. Further, whether the interventions would be cost-effective if it required significant health professional support in a long-run has not been documented well in the literature [33, 49]. Additional research with more time points of follow-up is warranted to maximize data to inform the compliance with the HITs, long-term impact on health outcomes, to look for evidence of harms and to determine the cost-effectiveness in the intervention [49]. Studies with CVD risk factor assessments and absolute outcome measurement are also needed.

Moreover, it is unknown which populations will benefit the most from the HIT intervention as the current research in HITs has not always directly engaged diverse end users. There are also many questions surrounding the "digital divide" in HITs use, where the access, usability, and effectiveness of diabetes technologies are divided by users' age, education, computer literacy, culture, and affluence [49]. These issues highlight the importance of engaging more research to design, test, and implement HITs for diverse patients with diabetes.

6. Barriers of using HITs in the real-world context and steps to move forward

While features of HITs can expand patients' ability in diabetes management and the results from the existing research showed their positive effects on outcomes of

HbA1c and CVD risk factors, many of these applications described above have so far been explored predominantly within clinical trials rather than a real-world context. For those that have been widely used in real health-care setting, such as electronic patient record system; both health-care providers and patients have reported difficulties for engagement [50]. Multiple sources of tension contribute to these barriers (**Table 2**).

First of all, the reliability and validity of some HITs is concerning. For example, many manufacturers market their products under the premise that they will help in improving health, but they often do not provide empirical evidence to support the effectiveness of their products [51]. Recent comparisons between different wearable devices for tracking physical activities yielded large heterogeneity in accuracy [52, 53]. The medical apps market also showed the similar discrepancy [54]. Lack of reliability is a serious obstacle that needs to be addressed before a HIT could be considered for medical use. Moreover, whether technological designs incorporated evidence-based guidelines is questionable [55]. It is reported that features of diabetes management apps on the online market did not cover evidence-based recommendations. A recent study evaluated 137 diabetes management apps from two major app stores (iTunes and Google Play) and compared the features with the American Association of Diabetes Educators (AADE) Self-Care Behavior guidelines. The author found an unbalanced feature development of current diabetes management apps. Few apps provided features supporting problem solving, reducing risks, and healthy coping, which are critical for user engagement and successful diabetes self-management [56].

Secondly, the privacy and security of personal data generated by HITs remains problematic. Users of these devices or technologies usually do not own the data; rather, data may be collected and stored by the manufacturers [51]. While some companies are willing to share user's "anonymizing" data via a simple distortion or removal of identifying features, these techniques do not provide adequate levels of anonymity and are not sufficient to prevent identity fraud [57]. Moreover, some devices are easily to be hacked as a result of various communication technologies that aid the transfer of data between the devices and smartphones. It has been reported that wireless digital pacemakers and glucose pumps are vulnerable to cyberattacks [58].

Further, even in relatively widely adopted HIT systems, such as the electronic patient records system, there are still many unfilled promises due to lack of interoperability between systems, difficult-to-use interface, and lack of consideration on patients' backgrounds [50]. In the United States, for example, the patient records

Barriers	Possible solutions
Validity and reliability	• Incorporating empirical evidence into design development • Being coherent with guidelines from credible sources • Evaluating users' needs and improve features on supporting problem solving, reducing risks, and healthy coping
Privacy and security	• Creating regulatory framework and risk-based classifications to promote innovation, protect patient safety, and avoid regulatory duplications
Adaptability	• Building interoperability between systems • Building easy-to-use interface • Providing incentives for engagement • Considering users' diverse background (language, health literacy, cultural preference)

Table 2.
Barriers of using HITs in the real-world context and possible solutions.

systems are not designed to talk to each other [59]. Until now, health-care providers have had little incentive to acquire or develop interoperable systems [50]. As a result, the current electronic health records do not allow a patient or provider to access needed health information anywhere at any time. Additionally, many clinicians are reluctant to invest the considerable time and effort to master difficult-to-use technology, which hindered the anticipated productivity gains of HITs [59]. Moreover, there are limited data collection on patient backgrounds, such as race/ethnicity, language preference, and health literacy in the patient records systems [49]. Lack of this set of data could cause fragmented care delivery and lead to patients' misunderstanding of provider instruction and lose trust in the medical system [49].

To transform HITs a real asset for diabetes care, further steps need to be considered (**Table 2**). First is to create a simple regulatory framework that does not suppress innovation but helps HITs, especially some wearable devices and apps become valid in the context of their health-oriented value [51]. A risk-based classification that promotes innovation, protects patient safety, and avoids regulatory duplications has recently been proposed [60]. As part of this model, the U.S. Food and Drug Administration jurisdiction covers higher-risk medical apps [61]. The National Health Service in the United Kingdom adopts similar pathway with their regulatory framework for mobile apps, which can be classified as "medical devices" by Medicines and Health Products Regulatory Agency [61].

A simple and powerful guide is also needed to transform the HIT system, especially the electronic patient records system. Health data stored in one system should be readily retrievable by others, subject to patient consent [50, 62]. For true interoperability, standardization must be achieved across three dimensions: how messages are sent and received; the structure and format of the information; and terms used within these dimensions [50]. HITs should also facilitate the work of clinicians by providing a system that is intuitive to use and without extensive retraining. Easy-to-use HIT systems not only will increase the productivity of providers but also will be safer [50].

Additionally, HIT systems need to include automated and standardized categories for a patient background (e.g., race/ethnicity, language), facilitate communication among multiple providers and patients, and tailor to the needs of diverse populations [9]. Moreover, a genuine partnership should be fostered between patients and health-care providers through the use of HITs. Engagement can range from patients being simply better informed to individuals themselves being dynamically engaged in the HIT management, giving feedbacks about the HIT interventions, and even controlling who has access to their data [62, 63]. Furthermore, future technologies developed for diabetes management should incorporate balanced features from creditable guidelines to better support changing self-management behaviors of people with diabetes.

7. Conclusion

Overall, the current evidence shows that HITs have favorable impact on glycemic control and CVD risk management among patients with T2D. Future studies should examine the long-term effects of HITs and their cost-effectiveness, potential harms, and test and verify their effectiveness in glycemic control and other important health indicators such as CVD risk factors, among diverse populations. HITs may be valuable tools in enhancing human health and well-being overall. However, their advances also pose challenges in aspects of validity and reliability, patients' privacy, security, and engagement. These issues need to be addressed before a broader implementation of HITs in the real-world setting.

Author details

Yilin Yoshida* and Eduardo J. Simoes
Department of Health Management and Informatics, School of Medicine,
University of Missouri-Columbia, Columbia, MO, USA

*Address all correspondence to: yoshiday@health.missouri.edu

References

[1] World Health Organization. Global Health Estimates 2016: Disease Burden by Cause, Age, Sex, by Country and by Region, 2000-2016. Geneva: World Health Organization; 2018

[2] Stratmann B, Tschoepe D. Heart in diabetes: Not only a macrovascular disease. Diabetes Care. 2011;**34** (Suppl 2):S138-S144

[3] Haffner SM, Lehto S, Ronnemaa T, Pyorala K, Laakso M. Mortality from coronary heart disease in subjects with type 2 diabetes and in nondiabetic subjects with and without prior myocardial infarction. The New England Journal of Medicine. 1998;**339**(4):229-234

[4] Lorber D. Importance of cardiovascular disease risk management in patients with type 2 diabetes mellitus. Diabetes, Metabolic Syndrome and Obesity. 2014;**7**:169-183

[5] Bujnowska-Fedak MM, Puchala E, Steciwko A. The impact of telehome care on health status and quality of life among patients with diabetes in a primary care setting in Poland. Telemedicine Journal and E-Health. 2011;**17**(3):153-163

[6] Bellazzi R, Arcelloni M, Bensa G, et al. Design, methods, and evaluation directions of a multi-access service for the management of diabetes mellitus patients. Diabetes Technology & Therapeutics. 2003;**5**(4):621-629

[7] Durso SC, Wendel I, Letzt AM, Lefkowitz J, Kaseman DF, Seifert RF. Older adults using cellular telephones for diabetes management: A pilot study. Medsurg Nursing. 2003;**12**(5):313-317

[8] Marchibroda JM. The impact of health information technology on collaborative chronic care management. Journal of Managed Care Pharmacy. 2008;**14**(2 Suppl):S3-S11

[9] Lopez L, Grant RW. Closing the gap: Eliminating health care disparities among Latinos with diabetes using health information technology tools and patient navigators. Journal of Diabetes Science and Technology. 2012;**6**(1):169-176

[10] Demiris G, Afrin LB, Speedie S, et al. Patient-centered applications: Use of information technology to promote disease management and wellness. A white paper by the AMIA knowledge in motion working group. Journal of the American Medical Informatics Association. 2008;**15**(1):8-13

[11] Jimison H, Gorman P, Woods S, et al. Barriers and drivers of health information technology use for the elderly, chronically ill, and underserved. Evidence Report/Technology Assessment. 2008;(175):1-1422

[12] Finkelstein J, O'Connor G, Friedmann RH. Development and implementation of the home asthma telemonitoring (HAT) system to facilitate asthma self-care. Studies in Health Technology and Informatics. 2001;**84**(Pt 1):810-814

[13] McTavish FM, Gustafson DH, Owens BH, et al. CHESS: An interactive computer system for women with breast cancer piloted with an under-served population. Proceedings of the Annual Symposium on Computer Applications in Medical Care. 1994:599-603. PMID: 7949998

[14] Veinot TC, Zheng K, Lowery JC, Souden M, Keith R. Using electronic health record Systems in diabetes care: Emerging practices. IHI. 2010;**2010**:240-249

[15] Milne RG, Horne M, Torsney B. SMS reminders in the UK national health service: An evaluation of its impact on "no-shows" at hospital out-patient clinics. Health Care Management Review. 2006;**31**(2):130-136

[16] Chung P, Yu T, Scheinfeld N. Using cellphones for teledermatology, a preliminary study. Dermatology Online Journal. 2007;**13**(3):2

[17] Weaver A, Young AM, Rowntree J, et al. Application of mobile phone technology for managing chemotherapy-associated side-effects. Annals of Oncology. 2007;**18**(11):1887-1892

[18] Tao D, Wang T, Wang T, Liu S, Qu X. Effects of consumer-oriented health information technologies in diabetes management over time: A systematic review and meta-analysis of randomized controlled trials. Journal of the American Medical Informatics Association. 2017;**24**(5):1014-1023

[19] Alharbi NS, Alsubki N, Jones S, Khunti K, Munro N, de Lusignan S. Impact of information technology-based interventions for type 2 diabetes mellitus on glycemic control: A systematic review and meta-analysis. Journal of Medical Internet Research. 2016;**18**(11):e310

[20] Faruque LI, Wiebe N, Ehteshami-Afshar A, et al. Effect of telemedicine on glycated hemoglobin in diabetes: A systematic review and meta-analysis of randomized trials. CMAJ. 2017;**189**(9):E341-E364

[21] Heitkemper EM, Mamykina L, Travers J, Smaldone A. Do health information technology self-management interventions improve glycemic control in medically underserved adults with diabetes? A systematic review and meta-analysis. Journal of the American Medical Informatics Association. 2017;**24**(5):1024-1035

[22] Marcolino MS, Maia JX, Alkmim MB, Boersma E, Ribeiro AL. Telemedicine application in the care of diabetes patients: Systematic review and meta-analysis. PLOS One. 2013;**8**(11):e79246

[23] Liang X, Wang Q, Yang X, et al. Effect of mobile phone intervention for diabetes on glycaemic control: A meta-analysis. Diabetic Medicine. 2011;**28**(4):455-463

[24] Pal K, Eastwood SV, Michie S, et al. Computer-based interventions to improve self-management in adults with type 2 diabetes: A systematic review and meta-analysis. Diabetes Care. 2014;**37**(6):1759-1766

[25] Costa BM, Fitzgerald KJ, Jones KM, Dunning Am T. Effectiveness of IT-based diabetes management interventions: A review of the literature. BMC Family Practice. 2009;**10**:72

[26] Rasekaba TM, Furler J, Blackberry I, Tacey M, Gray K, Lim K. Telemedicine interventions for gestational diabetes mellitus: A systematic review and meta-analysis. Diabetes Research and Clinical Practice. 2015;**110**(1):1-9

[27] Adaji A, Schattner P, Jones K. The use of information technology to enhance diabetes management in primary care: A literature review. Informatics in Primary Care. 2008;**16**(3):229-237

[28] Baron J, McBain H, Newman S. The impact of mobile monitoring technologies on glycosylated hemoglobin in diabetes: A systematic review. Journal of Diabetes Science and Technology. 2012;**6**(5):1185-1196

[29] Jaana M, Pare G. Home telemonitoring of patients with

diabetes: A systematic assessment of observed effects. Journal of Evaluation in Clinical Practice. 2007;**13**(2):242-253

[30] Marcolino AM, Barbosa RI, das Neves LM, Mazzer N, de Jesus Guirro RR, de Cassia Registro Fonseca M. Assessment of functional recovery of sciatic nerve in rats submitted to low-level laser therapy with different fluences. An experimental study: Laser in functional recovery in rats. Journal of Hand and Microsurgery. 2013;**5**(2):49-53

[31] Polisena J, Tran K, Cimon K, Hutton B, McGill S, Palmer K. Home telehealth for diabetes management: A systematic review and meta-analysis. Diabetes, Obesity & Metabolism. 2009;**11**(10):913-930

[32] Ramadas A, Quek KF, Chan CK, Oldenburg B. Web-based interventions for the management of type 2 diabetes mellitus: A systematic review of recent evidence. International Journal of Medical Informatics. 2011;**80**(6):389-405

[33] Yoshida Y, Boren SA, Soares J, et al. Current Diabetes Reports. 2018;**18**:130. https://doi.org/10.1007/s11892-018-1105-2

[34] Srimanunthiphol J, Beddow R, Arakaki R. A review of the United Kingdom prospective diabetes study (UKPDS) and a discussion of the implications for patient care. Hawaii Medical Journal. 2000;**59**(7):295, 313-298

[35] Sherifali D, Nerenberg K, Pullenayegum E, Cheng JE, Gerstein HC. The effect of oral antidiabetic agents on A1C levels: A systematic review and meta-analysis. Diabetes Care. 2010;**33**(8):1859-1864

[36] Choudhary P, Amiel SA. The use of technology to reduce hypoglycemia. Pediatric Endocrinology Reviews. 2010;**7**(Suppl 3):384-395

[37] Preis SR, Pencina MJ, Hwang SJ, et al. Trends in cardiovascular disease risk factors in individuals with and without diabetes mellitus in the Framingham heart study. Circulation. 2009;**120**(3):212-220

[38] Juutilainen A, Lehto S, Ronnemaa T, Pyorala K, Laakso M. Type 2 diabetes as a "coronary heart disease equivalent": An 18-year prospective population-based study in Finnish subjects. Diabetes Care. 2005;**28**(12):2901-2907

[39] Joseph J, Svartberg J, Njolstad I, Schirmer H. Change in cardiovascular risk factors in relation to diabetes status: The Tromso study. European Journal of Preventive Cardiology. 2012;**19**(3):551-557

[40] Saydah SH, Fradkin J, Cowie CC. Poor control of risk factors for vascular disease among adults with previously diagnosed diabetes. Journal of the American Medical Association. 2004;**291**(3):335-342

[41] Farkouh ME, Boden WE, Bittner V, et al. Risk factor control for coronary artery disease secondary prevention in large randomized trials. Journal of the American College of Cardiology. 2013;**61**(15):1607-1615

[42] Sieverdes JC, Treiber F, Jenkins C. Improving diabetes management with mobile health technology. The American Journal of the Medical Sciences. 2013;**345**(4):289-295

[43] eHealth Intiative. An Issue Brief on Health Information Technology and Cardiac Care; 2013

[44] Su D, Zhou J, Kelley MS, et al. Does telemedicine improve treatment outcomes for diabetes? A meta-analysis of results from 55 randomized controlled trials. Diabetes Research and Clinical Practice. 2016;**116**:136-148

[45] Pal K, Eastwood SV, Michie S, et al. Computer-based diabetes

self-management interventions for adults with type 2 diabetes mellitus. Cochrane Database of Systematic Reviews. 2013;**3**:CD008776

[46] Krantz DS, Baum A, Wideman M. Assessment of preferences for self-treatment and information in health care. Journal of Personality and Social Psychology. 1980;**39**(5):977-990

[47] Goyder C, McPherson A, Glasziou P. Diagnosis in general practice. Self diagnosis. BMJ. 2009;**339**:b4418

[48] O'Kane MJ, Bunting B, Copeland M, Coates VE, Es Group. Efficacy of self monitoring of blood glucose in patients with newly diagnosed type 2 diabetes (ESMON study): Randomised controlled trial. BMJ. 2008;**336**(7654):1174-1177

[49] Lopez L, Green AR, Tan-McGrory A, King R, Betancourt JR. Bridging the digital divide in health care: The role of health information technology in addressing racial and ethnic disparities. Joint Commission Journal on Quality and Patient Safety. 2011;**37**(10):437-445

[50] Kellermann AL, Jones SS. What it will take to achieve the as-yet-unfulfilled promises of health information technology. Health Affairs. 2013;**32**(1):63-68

[51] Piwek L, Ellis DA, Andrews S, Joinson A. The rise of consumer health wearables: Promises and barriers. PLoS Medicine. 2016;**13**(2):e1001953

[52] Lee JM, Kim Y, Welk GJ. Validity of consumer-based physical activity monitors. Medicine and Science in Sports and Exercise. 2014;**46**(9):1840-1848

[53] Case MA, Burwick HA, Volpp KG, Patel MS. Accuracy of smartphone applications and wearable devices for tracking physical activity data. Journal of the American Medical Association. 2015;**313**(6):625-626

[54] Wolf JA, Moreau JF, Akilov O, et al. Diagnostic inaccuracy of smartphone applications for melanoma detection. JAMA Dermatology. 2013;**149**(4):422-426

[55] Chomutare T, Fernandez-Luque L, Arsand E, Hartvigsen G. Features of mobile diabetes applications: Review of the literature and analysis of current applications compared against evidence-based guidelines. Journal of Medical Internet Research. 2011;**13**(3):e65

[56] Ye Q, Khan U, Boren SA, Simoes EJ, Kim MS. An analysis of diabetes mobile applications features compared to AADE7: Addressing self-management behaviors in people with diabetes. Journal of Diabetes Science and Technology. 2018;**12**(4):808-816

[57] Kosinski M, Stillwell D, Graepel T. Private traits and attributes are predictable from digital records of human behavior. Proceedings of the National Academy of Sciences of the United States of America. 2013;**110**(15):5802-5805

[58] Maisel WH, Kohno T. Improving the security and privacy of implantable medical devices. The New England Journal of Medicine. 2010;**362**(13):1164-1166

[59] O'Malley AS, Grossman JM, Cohen GR, Kemper NM, Pham HH. Are electronic medical records helpful for care coordination? Experiences of physician practices. Journal of General Internal Medicine. 2010;**25**(3):177-185

[60] Cortez NG, Cohen IG, Kesselheim AS. FDA regulation of mobile health technologies. The New England Journal of Medicine. 2014;**371**(4):372-379

[61] McCartney M. How do we know whether medical apps work? BMJ. 2013;**346**:f1811

[62] Kreitmair KV, Cho MK, Magnus DC. Consent and engagement, security, and authentic living using wearable and mobile health technology. Nature Biotechnology. 2017;**35**(7):617-620

[63] Wilbanks J, Friend SH. First, design for data sharing. Nature Biotechnology. 2016;**34**(4):377-379